Meditation for Psychot

Meditation for Psychotherapists provides students and practitioners of psychotherapy with specific meditation techniques.

Chapters offer a comprehensive theoretical and practical approach as an adjunct to established professional development tools. This is the first time specific bespoke meditation techniques have been connected to different therapeutic modalities, building on the author's already published work.

The book is accompanied by a website with audio-guided meditations and courses directed to an international audience across multiple psychotherapy models www.arosspsychotherapy.com/meditation.

Alexander H. Ross is a psychodynamic psychotherapist working in the NHS and private practice in London.

"Psychological therapies have enormous potential to alleviate suffering and transform people's lives. But they depend on psychological therapists who are both skilled and resourced to do this important and challenging work. Research tells us which therapies are effective and regardless of therapy modality that the therapist is important. This book seeks to resource therapists with mindfulness; more than this to match specific meditation techniques to therapeutic modalities.

With clarity, deep subject knowledge and a wealth of experience, this book sets out how mindfulness can support therapists in their work. Recognising that therapists bring themselves to work, Dr Ross explains how mindfulness can support their effectiveness, but also ensure they are nourished to do the work.

The book is imbued with three interwoven strands that together give it its strength. First, Dr Ross is an experienced therapist, and draws on a wealth of experience that brings the book to life and lends it humanity. Second, he walks the talk of clarity, compassion, courage, and a sense of optimism about psychotherapeutic work. Third, he draws together a deep understanding of both therapy and Buddhism. Finally, he weaves these strands together masterfully into a compelling and powerful weft.

Several research studies suggest that therapists who learn mindfulness do better personally and professionally. This is a book any therapist with an interest in mindfulness should read to enrich their work."

Willem Kuyken, *Ritblat Professor of Mindfulness and Psychological Science, University of Oxford*

"Mindfulness has gained great popularity in recent years, but few seem to dive deeply into other types of meditation. Dr Alexander Ross has put together a marvelously broad overview of many forms of meditation and how they relate to the various schools of psychotherapy. Providing more than just academic descriptions, Dr Ross expresses insights from the depth of his own personal practice. Highly recommended for those who would like to integrate their psychotherapy with sophisticated meditation practices, complete with scripts and questions to process the exercises."

Richard Jishou Sears, *PsyD, psychologist, Zen master, and author of* Mindfulness: Living Through Challenges and Enriching Your Life in This Moment

"With clarity and precision, Dr Ross deftly blends together Western psychology, neuroscience, physiology, and meditation practices, creating a superb guide for mental health practitioners looking to understand and use meditation as a clinical anchor and ally. The volume is a remarkable addition to the ongoing important dialogue between Western therapeutic approaches and the timeless wisdom of contemplative practices."

Fiona Brandon, *MA, MFT, contemplative psychotherapist and co-editor of* Advances in Contemplative Psychotherapy

Meditation for Psychotherapists

Targeted Techniques to Enhance Your Clinical Skills

Alexander H. Ross

Routledge
Taylor & Francis Group

NEW YORK AND LONDON

Designed cover image: © MarinMtk Getty Images

First published 2025
by Routledge
605 Third Avenue, New York, NY 10158

and by Routledge
4 Park Square, Milton Park, Abingdon, Oxon, OX14 4RN

Routledge is an imprint of the Taylor & Francis Group, an informa business

Library of Congress Cataloging-in-Publication Data
Names: Ross, Alexander H., author.
Title: Meditation for psychotherapists : targeted techniques to enhance
your clinical skills / Alexander H. Ross.
Description: New York, NY : Routledge, 2025. | Includes bibliographical
references and index.
Identifiers: LCCN 2024025423 (print) | LCCN 2024025424 (ebook) |
ISBN 9781032453507 (hardback) | ISBN 9781032453514 (paperback) |
ISBN 9781003382959 (ebook)
Subjects: LCSH: Meditation--Therapeutic use.
Classification: LCC RC489.M43 R66 2025 (print) |
LCC RC489.M43 (ebook) | DDC 158.1/28--dc23/eng/20240614
LC record available at https://lccn.loc.gov/2024025423
LC ebook record available at https://lccn.loc.gov/2024025424

ISBN: 978-1-032-45350-7 (hbk)
ISBN: 978-1-032-45351-4 (pbk)
ISBN: 978-1-003-38295-9 (ebk)

DOI: 10.4324/9781003382959

Typeset in Palatino
by KnowledgeWorks Global Ltd.

Contents

Preface

For the past fifteen years, I have regularly been on meditation retreats, usually silent, that might last for a day, a weekend or up to ten days. It was on one of these retreats, while I was training as a psychotherapist, that the idea which forms this book first came into my mind. At the time, I wasn't aware that it would grow to become the book I have written. Indeed, by the end of the retreat, I had actually forgotten the idea and it took a fair few months for it to bubble back up into my consciousness, a frustrating time as I knew I was onto something interesting, but for the life of me I couldn't recall exactly what it was. The idea started because on this particular ten-day retreat, a range of meditation techniques were practised. The first was for the purpose of generating concentration, then using that concentration to explore the impermanent constantly changing nature of the mind, body and external reality, followed by a meditation on goodwill to leave the retreat feeling more comfortable. At the time, the idea which emerged was that just as different meditation techniques had been taught which developed concentration, discernment or goodwill, in the same way, a specific meditation practice could be used to develop the different states of mind that a therapist has in the type of psychodynamic psychotherapy in which I was training. The idea fortunately returned to me, which was a great relief, akin to finally being able to finally vocalise something which is on the end of one's tongue.

I think back now and speculate that until that point, I had always separated these two parts of my life – psychotherapy and meditation, both in their own ways, trainings that seek to develop certain characteristics. I think now that I had perhaps been worried that one might negate or challenge the other, so I had unconsciously forgotten my idea of bringing them closer together. The more I have worked on this, the more I have found that if approached in a particular way, each can actually enhance the other. My meditation practice is now as important to my psychotherapy work as supervision or other continuous professional development work.

Freud's concept of evenly suspended attention and the use of countertransference in the British object relations school both lent themselves well to this idea. It is these thoughts which will provide some of the content for two of the chapters. After publishing an initial paper making these connections (Ross, 2021), I then thought about different therapy modalities, which might also describe a state of mind the practitioner embodies and how other meditation techniques in which I had trained may be suited for them.

When I looked to see if this idea had been presented before, I found that, in general, off-the-peg meditation techniques, usually Zen Buddhist or secular mindfulness meditations, had been used by therapists looking to enhance their robustness, receptivity or connection with clients in quite a general way. Various trials and studies using these types of meditation techniques will be explored in the section on *The Current Evidence Base*. There had also been much written comparing various psychotherapy modalities with other spiritual, often Buddhist traditions, sometimes, but not always with a chapter on a general meditation that could support a psychotherapist in their work. What I hope to add is to show how particular states of mind can be developed with certain meditations that can match a specific psychotherapy modality and the mindset that a therapist might have when practising that therapy model.

I have also developed and taught meditation courses to students training as medical professionals for them to better manage the stress of their roles. Through this, I have gained experience in how best to approach beginners and which methods and explanations are most helpful to support others to develop an enthusiasm for meditation, which I hope this book will go some way to support across the psychotherapy community. While there has been a strong focus on using meditation as a therapeutic modality in itself, I hope that this book will show how it can be a powerful adjunct to established methods of training, which will be more familiar to readers. I know in my own development as a clinician, meditation has been invaluable to support my own work, both for myself and my clients and I am keen to share this.

I think it is important to acknowledge that while I have what I believe to be necessary experience in both meditation and psychotherapy to speak with some expertise on the topics, I am also approaching what has been a relatively recent import to my own culture – be that professionally in psychotherapy, or speaking from a wider cultural perspective. I am conscious of this as I attempt to integrate two culturally different practices and I hope I am treating both with necessary sensitivity within this context with the awareness of where I am an insider addressing outsiders, but also vice versa. I am deeply indebted to those traditions from which I have and continue to learn, none more so than the Buddhist tradition of Thai Forest Theravada that I most identify with in my beliefs and practice. I hope that this book can aid in more integration and stimulate thought amongst places that may have seemed historically and culturally quite separate and potentially at odds with each other without denuding either of the meanings that are integral to their identity.

I am particularly enthusiastic about the benefits of meditating with others and how that enhances practice. In the spirit of this, I will be offering in-person and online courses for therapists to gain more experience and confidence in their meditation practice as well as share their experiences to develop this field. You can find out more about guided meditations and opportunities for meditation courses both online and in person on my website www.arosspsychotherapy.com/meditation.

References

Ross, A. (2021). On meditation and the development of the internal analytic setting. *British Journal of Psychotherapy*, 38(1), pp.98–115.

Acknowledgements

I'm extremely grateful to my family for their patience and loving support while I wrote this book, encouraging me through the many ups, downs and moments of self-doubt. I'm deeply indebted to the therapists who have supported me, the clients from whom I have learned, the fellow meditators I have sat with and the meditation teachers who have guided me over many years. I would like to thank Anne Jennings for her enthusiasm and support when I first embarked on writing about meditation and psychotherapy, and Dr Karen Treisman for her assistance when approaching my publishers with the initial concept for this book. I'd like to also extend my gratitude for specific guidance from colleagues – Alex Kidd for giving me advice about all things mentalisation-based, Alia Butt for illuminating me about phenomenology and everything existential, and Joshua Marks for his help in bringing the book to publication.

About the Author

Dr Alexander Ross trained and practised as a medical doctor before qualifying as a psychodynamic psychotherapist at the Tavistock and has over a decade's experience working with people in mental distress. Dr Ross currently works as a psychotherapist in an NHS acute crisis service and in private practice in London, UK. Dr Ross has been meditating for fifteen years with a range of different approaches, finding his home in the Thai Forest Buddhist tradition.

Introduction

In the first instance, this book will serve as a complete introductory text for therapists of different modalities to understand what meditation is and how it can be used to complement their clinical skills. I say introductory as there will be a foundation of theory and evidence, the practicalities of how to learn and train as a meditator, how to bring the techniques into the therapy room and ways to manage common and uncommon difficulties that arise. However, it is the practice itself, which, of course, will occur beyond the reading of this book, that will support a meditator to take this introduction into their clinical work. I feel it is complete as it holds all the information, which I believe to work as an introductory guide aside from the actual practice, which comes from the meditators themselves. It is made for both therapists in training and qualified, anyone interested in the connections between different therapy modalities and meditation traditions or who has an interest in meditation and how it might be helpful in this specific area, which I feel has until now been under-investigated with literature scattered within different books and published papers. In addition to therapists, other healthcare professionals who work in the field of mental health, such as psychologists, psychiatrists and social workers, will also find elements of the book useful and I'm sure, would have much to gain from a meditation practice that aligns itself with the mindset with which they work. This book brings together and makes explicit the connections between meditation and psychotherapy practice so that you can understand how each can complement the other.

While I describe different therapy modalities and match specific techniques to them, I don't want readers to imagine that, therefore, they should only be practising that particular technique. To that end, in the latter part of the book I will describe other methods that might be helpful for any person practising as a therapist, or not even a therapist. I would also urge you to look through the whole book, as while it might be tempting to jump to your own particular model of clinical practice, each chapter builds on the previous and I have left some of the more challenging practices to the latter chapters of the book.

I also hope that you will approach the book with an open mind. There's no getting away from the fact that meditation has its own cultural and religious associations. For this reason, I have been particular in my use of language. I have selected meditation rather than mindfulness to separate these practices from those which are more familiar to us as therapeutic techniques and so it can have as broad a definition as possible incorporating a range of different methods beyond secular mindfulness meditation. I will go into more detail about the history and reasons behind this in the *What About Mindfulness?* section. However, I am aware that in doing so, the idea of meditation comes with its own relationship and associations with religious and spiritual traditions which someone who has a more scientific background might find alienating.

While I have mostly trained within religious traditions spending varying amounts of time in Zen, Vajrayana and Theravada Buddhist communities and retreats as well as a Hare Krishna community, I will be keeping things secular and when possible related to scientific concepts in the fields of psychology, neuroscience and physiology so as to ensure as many people as possible can relate to the book. However, there will also be some explanations that I think of as more metaphorical or symbolic, which might be closer to those spiritual descriptions that others might find more meaningful. That said, I want to demystify meditation and take it a step away from what can often appear to be more magical thinking, but equally give you an opportunity to take the full potential of benefits from it when sometimes it can be presented in quite a limited and cold way. There might be aspects with which you disagree, but I hope you will be able to temporarily park some of these disagreements to find a meditation practice which resonates. I am, of course, looking forward to engaging with the full range of reactions that I expect this book will bring forth.

I often think it's helpful to approach meditation with two mindsets:

♦ A Scientist – to test hypotheses, discard those which do not work and converge on a hypothesis and practice which fulfils the goal of developing in whichever way you would like as a clinician and
♦ An Explorer – to seek out and discover new and different ways to practise outside of your usual experience, working with an open mind in potentially unfamiliar ways, reserving judgement until the full extent of the practice has been understood.

Everyone will approach this book with their own set of experiences and as such, not all the techniques will be useful or maybe even appropriate for them due to previous meditation or other experiences, concentration levels at a given time, time available for practice and many other personal and environmental reasons. In many meditation traditions there is the idea of what I call the one true path – that there is the one and only technique that will work to deliver whatever outcome the practitioner is hoping, often carrying the implication that others are inferior. I am not of this opinion, and I think that keeping in mind these two roles as scientist and explorer will allow you to discover which techniques are best for you at a given time or place without feeling too alienated by the techniques that may not resonate or may not be possible at that particular point or state.

I will start the book by describing my understanding of what meditation is. This is informed mostly by my own practice across many different meditation traditions for the past fifteen years. I will also be using some of the language which has been adapted from the work of Thanissaro Bikkhu (Geoffrey DeGraff), a Buddhist monk and scholar. Thanissaro Bikkhu has translated early Buddhist texts from the original Pali into English taking special care to pick appropriate words that express the meaning of these mental processes most accurately (Thanissaro, 2012). I find them clear, logical, closely related to my own experiences and adaptable to show connections with different psychotherapies.

I have used personal meditation experiences and my psycho-therapy training and practice to adapt this work and to show equivalents and overlaps with terms in psychotherapy. I have used these terms to develop what I call a meditation framework through which a range of techniques can then be attached. I will follow this with the evidence base that has been established, showing how meditation is useful for therapists as well as the limitations of the techniques employed in this research.

Each chapter will then map out the different mindsets required for a range of psychotherapy modalities and one or more corresponding meditation techniques. The different models – psychoanalytic or psychodynamic psychotherapy, body-centred psychotherapies, person-centred counselling, mentalisation-based therapy and existential therapy have all been chosen as they have a specific description of the mindset which the therapist has when in the consultation room with clients. I will be describing this as the internal setting which I think encompasses the full range of this mindset – how it relates to the therapist themselves as well as in relation to the client. I recognise that there is a certain emphasis on the psychodynamic approach and language in the book which comes from my own specific training and experience which I hope will not alienate readers who are not so familiar with this. I have made extra efforts to explain any technical language so that readers from academic or non-clinical backgrounds will be able to follow the concepts and practices. If a reader practices another psychotherapy modality not mentioned in the book, I have no doubt that they too will still find overlaps with their own way of working due to the range of methods mentioned.

In each chapter, I will describe the internal setting for that specific therapy and map a different meditation technique onto it using the meditation framework. At the end of each chapter, there will be a full description of the technique with an accom-panying audio recording of a guided meditation allowing you to practise yourself by listening along to this having read the explanation in the book. I recognise that many therapists work with a range of modalities in an integrative way and might like some other general techniques to draw on, so I end the book with some other meditation techniques that I think complement those already presented. When describing each method, I will make connections and references to neuroscientific, physiological or psychological theories to help inform my reasoning for suggesting a specific meditation technique. I will end with a chapter on *Troubleshooting* addressing many of the difficulties that arise when meditating and ways I've found to be effective in countering them.

Different psychotherapy traditions use a range of language to describe the therapist and the person who comes to see them. I realise that some prefer counsellor, therapist or psychotherapist and patient, client or service user – each word with its own advantages, disadvantages, historical context and perspective. To keep things as broad as possible, I will be sticking to using the nomenclature of the therapist and client.

Thinking more broadly, I consider meditation a countercultural activity. Increasingly, the commodity being exchanged for supposedly free technological products is our time, but maybe more accurately our attention. Technological developments also often sell themselves as increasing efficiency but ultimately may be a drain on our internal resources and capacity for meaningful interpersonal and internal relationships. Through meditation practice, we aim to develop a stronger internal awareness and correspondingly a more considered attention. This can serve as a counterbalance to the sometimes overwhelming and highly addictive presence of technology.

Meditation also offers an opportunity for us to challenge concepts around self-identity and fixed belief systems. In recent years, society has had an increasing focus on the self through social media encouraging and emphasising self-censorship and external monitoring, which is highly encouraging of conformity. In addition, our identities are often built up around external displays of what we consume, both by algorithms designed to sell us more of these items and those to group people together with similar profiles. Meditation can offer us a perspective to peel away and bring to light some of these layers by helping us to notice that there is more flexibility and plasticity in aspects of identity and ourselves than might be initially apparent. This might seem paradoxical as meditation, being inward gazing, could be perceived as another method of bolstering self-identity. This will be explored more in the *Responding to Criticisms* section of the book, but in brief, meditation, much like psychotherapy, can result in changes in the way we think about ourselves through greater self-understanding. Meditation can contribute to insights into how our experience of reality is potentially more self-constructed than we may realise on an everyday level, releasing ourselves from constraints and conventional understandings of more fixed identities and beliefs that may hold us back from bringing about change.

While I present this book as a complete introduction, I also want to establish the limits and boundaries of my expounding meditation as what I feel to be an important part of my work as a psychotherapist. As mentioned before, I don't believe there is one true path in terms of meditation techniques. Likewise, I don't think there is one true path in psychotherapy modalities. While I hope after reading and practising meditation, you may put it in the same category of importance as other training methods, I would not wish to suggest that it is here to replace these methods. Rather, I hope it complements established approaches. As far as reading this book and applying it independently can set a foundation for understanding and practice, I also want to emphasise that this can only get one so far. Meditating with others, especially with the guidance of a teacher preferably in person, but if not online, not only offers bespoke direction, but being around others also working in a similar way will help to further the establishment of a meditation habit greatly. I'm sure this is a familiar concept for those of you who have been through psychotherapy training, which would be impossible to do without the guidance of a supervisor and challenging without the support of peers. I also believe that the embodied presence of in-person work is superior to online because meditation is a mind and body experience and therefore, to be physically with others is preferable. I am aware, however, that this is not an opinion entirely shared by others and that online is definitely better than nothing. Research shows that lifetime persistence in a meditation practice is enhanced by having spoken with a teacher but is negatively associated with initial exposure through technology or due to mental health issues (Lam et al., 2023). So, beginning with a book and then perhaps attending a course or retreat may be a good foundation for the onward development of meditation practice.

Chapter Summary

♦ The book will serve as a complete introductory text for psychotherapists or anyone working in the field of mental health to develop a meditation practice

♦ There will be general meditation methods described and also ones specific to certain psychotherapy modalities

♦ There will be explanations throughout the book from the fields of psychology, neuroscience, physiology and more metaphorical perspectives

♦ Readers should approach the practice with the mindset of both an explorer and a scientist to find out what works best for them

♦ Meditation has a wider cultural context and potential for change beyond our professional lives

♦ Development can be supported by meditating with a group and working with a teacher.

References

Lam, S.U., Riordan, K.M., Simonsson, O., Davidson, R.J. and Goldberg, S.B. (2023). Who sticks with meditation? Rates and predictors of persistence in a population-based sample in the USA. *Mindfulness*, 14, pp.66–68.

Thanissaro, B. (2012). *Right Mindfulness, Memory and Ardency on the Buddhist Path*. California, USA: Metta Forest Monastery.

1 Introduction to Meditation

The Meditation Framework

Meditation is a practice which uses a specific type of awareness to develop the qualities of:

- **Concentration** – attention on a specific object. This can be on a range between either focussed or open concentration
- **Discernment** – the ability to make an informed judgement about the object under the spotlight of this attention. This can be on a range between either evaluating or non-judgemental discernment.

To this end, the practice utilises and refines three types of awareness loosely structured around the time continuum:

Past – mindfulness: Recalling the meditation object and remembering to keep it in mind

Present – alertness or comprehension: Awareness of what is happening, noticing what you are doing and focussed on currently

Future – ardency, keenness and effort: The desire and motivation to take up skilful and abandon unskilful mental qualities (these qualities are defined as skilful by whether they support the development of the desired end results of concentration and discernment around the meditation object).

DOI: 10.4324/9781003382959-1

The techniques in this book will use a range of primary objects for this awareness generally starting with breath – meditation techniques also commonly known as breathwork – but also meditation objects encompassing other bodily sensations, feelings, thoughts as well as using the imagination and visualisations. Each meditation technique will help to develop a specific mindset which, once developed, can then be brought to the consulting room to enhance your ability to be able to work with a client in whichever modality you work by making the internal setting more readily accessible as well as improving resilience, robustness and presence with a client. There will be suggestions for other techniques that can be utilised immediately before, during and after meeting with clients.

Comparisons can be made between different meditation techniques by showing where they sit on ranges between the three variables outlined above to display the mental qualities developed from a given meditation practice:

1. **Concentration:** Open awareness ←→ Focussed awareness
2. **Discernment:** Evaluating awareness ←→ Non-judgemental awareness
3. **Time continuum:** Remembering/mindfulness ←→ Present/ alertness ←→ Future/ardency.

Meditation exists on a range between these metrics with difference styles placed at different points. The technique of a given meditation can help to develop one of these more than the other. For example, in the concentration range, you can be particularly focussed on an object such as the breath by using alertness and comprehension of the present moment and mindfulness to repeatedly return awareness to the breath when it wanders. By only concentrating on the breath, or even one particular part of the breath such as the tip of the nose, you have a focussed instead of open awareness and are more evaluating than non-judgemental by noticing other experiences that arise in other sensory modalities and abandoning focus on them in exchange for greater concentration on the object. This is a useful mental quality when listening intently to what and how a client is talking. This technique would be more evaluating and focussed, utilising alertness and mindfulness.

On the evaluating to non-judgemental awareness range of discernment, an awareness which notices and accepts the breath and any other arising phenomena without consciously changing them would place it firmly on the non-judgemental side. In terms of concentration, it would be more of an open awareness. This mental quality supports the clinical approach of a more accepting state of mind which absorbs what a client may be saying without conscious judgement and waits for ideas and feelings to emerge from the therapist's unconscious. One perhaps more akin to Rogerian therapy which will be more fully described in the chapter on *Person-Centred Counselling*.

However, if a more evaluating awareness was chosen whereby the breath was altered in order to change the experience, a more discerning and less non-judgemental state of mind can be developed. This employs more ardency to take up a different way to change the breath to establish a consequential change in the state of mind. This conscious evaluation and reassessment of the object renders a mental quality which can be helpful to make a more conscious analysis of what a client may be expressing to the therapist and can be helpful to support a more discerning internal therapeutic setting.

It is recognised that too much of any of the metrics could be unhelpful, and having the flexibility to move between them is often desirable. These ranges therefore are a useful way to point towards mental qualities, but the actual experience of these is more ineffable and understood through practice. These examples will also make more sense once they can be attached to descriptions of internal settings in later chapters. That is why this book isn't just a list of meditation techniques but attaches them to certain internal settings and psychotherapy modalities.

Therefore, using the meditation framework, we follow the instructions of mindfulness – remembering the focus of the meditation and bringing our minds back to it, alertness – trying to stay on the meditation object in the present moment and also using ardency – putting effort into taking up the aims of the meditation and letting go of those that might get in the way or take things in a different direction. So perhaps in a meditation method for developing the state of mind in person-centred counselling we would be generating a sense of unconditional positive regard and reducing feelings of being judgemental and trying to change the way a client is. This then produces the specific state of mind in terms of concentration and discernment, allows for thoughts that are helpful and then gets away from the idea of simply not thinking. In essence, we are giving ourselves something to do to focus on a way of being, emerging through the process of meditation.

As for the development of these internal settings, in fact, the real fruits of meditation are realised outside of the meditation itself. An analogy is that meditation is like learning to drive in a car park or parking lot. No matter how good one is at parallel parking with plenty of time and space, the skill is not really tested or developed until it is attempted with another car waiting and only a cramped space available. Likewise, reality testing the results of meditation is crucial, in this case that would be in the consultation room, but the benefits of meditation are wide-ranging, and if practised regularly, you will notice a host of physical and psychological benefits occurring professionally, but also in everyday life.

Other Classifications and Definitions of Meditation

This book is different to most meditation guides in that we will take a description of a specific mindset before mapping a meditation technique onto that. Generally, the technique itself is the starting point of most meditation books, or if it is from a spiritual or religious perspective, then it shows how a meditation technique might be attached to a certain belief system or way of life. The latter might be closer to here, where instead of a belief or lifestyle, the starting point is a certain psychotherapy modality. Often, one specific mindset might be applied to a range of techniques. For example, an open, non-judgemental, present-moment awareness is brought to observing the breath, feelings of compassion or a body scan. In traditions where one technique reigns supreme, this might be the source of multiple mindsets. For example, the technique might be breath meditation and the mindsets being different degrees of focus and insight into the connection between mind and body, and how this can be perceived as being created and therefore altered ultimately from the mind. In this book, technique and mindset are closely bound together, each influencing the other. The following classification systems are not exhaustive, but all offer different perspectives on how to think about the myriad of different approaches to meditation.

One approach to classifying meditation has been to take a *bottom-up approach* using 100 meditators to rate and combine similarities of the 20 most previously established popular techniques, trimmed down from an initial list of 309 techniques:

> Based on our results, we propose a two-dimensional system of classifying meditation according to (1) the amount of body orientation in the technique, and (2) the level of activation in the technique. Furthermore, we propose seven main clusters of meditation techniques, namely: (1) Body-centered meditation, (2) mindful observation, (3) contemplation, (4) mantra meditation, (5) visual concentration, (6) affect-centered meditation, and (7) meditation with movement.
>
> (Matko and Sedlmeier, 2019)

Another approach has been to create a phenomenological classification of mindfulness meditation in an attempt to bring together the huge array of experiences that meditators have that are sometimes all classified together as one monolithic mindfulness block (Lutz et al., 2015). The researchers present meditation across three different dimensions:

1. Object orientation – the experience of a mental state being directed towards a certain object;
2. Dereification – whether thoughts, feelings and perceptions are regarded as mental processes rather than more objective representations of external reality and
3. Meta-awareness – that state of turning the attention and noticing the state of consciousness.

There are then four secondary dimensions:

1. Aperture – the degree that attention is focussed
2. Clarity – the vividness of this attention
3. Stability – how much the experience persists and
4. Effort – how easy this can be maintained.

Criticisms of these two classifications include that the former does not incorporate techniques which are not embodied, such as those involving deep states of concentration, and the latter only involves the systems known under the umbrella of mindfulness meditation. They also do not include other important details of meditation methods (MMs), including different postures, the degree to which eyes are open or closed or where attention might be focussed on specific body regions (Sparby and Sacchet, 2022). I think this set of issues might be more directed to the first system proposed. The second is more about the meditator's experience or mindset, as I call it in this book, rather than the focus of the technique. However, it is true that these points aren't incorporated. Therefore, Sparby and Sacchet propose an integrated model incorporating the context – spiritual or secular, the intention or motivation and then the practice itself – involving the degree of effort, the connection between activity and consequential effect, and how formal this practice is. There is also a clear differentiation between whether a technique is active or receptive. The researchers conclude with a definition of meditation as an attempt to rectify the above criticisms and provide a description that is neither too broad nor narrow:

> Meditation is at least one of several intentional awareness activities such as observe, focus, release, produce, imagine, and move, underpinned and unified by the activity of awareness of awareness, performed in a formal or informal setting. The practice of these activities may result in altered states of consciousness, passing through stages of development, and ultimately endpoints of practices (e.g., "awakening," "enlightenment") (Reddy and Roy, 2019). These states, stages, and experiences (or lack of

experience) may be motivated by and interpreted within secular or spiritual frameworks.

(Sparby and Sacchet, 2022)

In order to take a more empirical and neuroscientific approach, another method has been to review studies involving meditation and fMRI (functional magnetic resonance imagery) – a type of brain scan which measures blood flow in the brain corresponding to activity levels in those specific areas (Engström, Willander and Simon, 2021). They looked at 28 studies scanning meditators performing a range of meditation techniques. Four themes were identified:

1. The present moment
2. Wholesome qualities to cultivate
3. Unwholesome qualities to avoid
4. Attitudes

Covering four domains of brain function:

1. Cognitive
2. Affective
3. Somatic
4. Self

This provides a very broad set of categories that probably miss quite a lot of nuance between techniques and various elements of practice. However, as derived from MRI scans, it provides a useful system for future research from a neurological perspective as it has a foundation in the specific connections between brain function and meditation.

An approach to integrate the problem of the range of experiences and techniques has been to utilise a classification system based on taxonomy and systematics (the study of biodiversity) backed up by neuroscientific findings (Nash and Newberg, 2013, 2023) of which by definition, the authors found the above classification systems did not satisfy. In order to develop criteria, the intention or directionality of the technique

was selected rather than the less easily defined phenomenological perspective, longer-term goals or specific techniques.
The result is a comprehensive three-tier system, which I think
resolves the limitations of the other classifications above. The
first tier divides the MMs into simple and complex. The simple
methods are separated into three categories:

1. Affective directed methods – associated with developing
   different effects such as the method described in the
   chapter on *Person-Centred Counselling – Unconditional
   Positive Regard*;
2. Cognitive directed methods – associated with developing
   different cognitive states, such as the method described
   in the section on *Evenly Suspended Attention* and
3. Null directed methods – associated with developing neither a cognitive nor affective state, such as the chapter on
   without memory or desire and negative capability.

The complex methods are divided into four types that combine the simple methods:

1. Affective and cognitive
2. Affective and null
3. Cognitive and null
4. All three

The *Establishing The Meditation Frame* method, which I use as
the foundation for all the other techniques, would probably fall
into complex type 1 and when developed further in the *Breathing
Throughout The Body* method found in the *Other Complementary
Techniques* chapter becomes a complex type 4 method. I find the complex type 2 and 3 categories a bit harder to see how the techniques
I propose fit. The authors of the paper only suggest one technique,
which is more than two techniques practised consequentially.
Therefore, nearly all of the meditations I present would fall into the
complex category as I suggest readers to first *establish the meditation
frame* before embarking on another method. Aside from this issue,
it seems to cover all the potential methods I have in the book.

The third tier of classification goes into much more detail in nine categories in order to classify all the different details of the MMs that coexist within one domain:

1. The specific cognitive strategies which are prescribed within the MM directions (what one has to do in order to achieve the intended result) e.g., concentration/focused attention, passive observation without attachment, visualization and imagination, memorization and repetition, selective or effortless awareness, contemplation, introspection, inquiry, sensory perception(s)…

2. The conceptual and/or physical object(s) that are the focus of attention e.g., the breath, a mantra, a symbol, an image, a phrase, an idea, a narrative, a sound, etc. …

3. Whether the MM (meditation method) requires certain beliefs or special knowledge, i.e., a particular religious, spiritual, metaphysical, or philosophical teaching or system. …

4. Whether the MM requires that the eyes remain closed or open, and if particular eye movements are prescribed. …

5. Whether the process requires a relatively static position or certain kinetic elements. Here "static" refers to a stationary body but not necessarily an immobile body, e.g., bodily movements occur but the body still remains essentially in one place, as when the meditator changes postures from an upright sitting position to a more reclined position, or experiences involuntary jerking motions. "Kinetic" refers to prescribed movements of the body such as movements of the extremities as in walking meditation, Tai Chi, and mudras (hand movements). …

6. Whether the process is non-verbal (silent/sub-vocal), verbal (vocal), or both. …

7. Whether a specific type of postural position is suggested or required, e.g., seated in a normal comfortable position, straight spine, lotus position, fully reclined, supine, or standing (this key could be considered as a sub-set of #5 above). …

8. Whether the process is intrinsic (self-reliant/independent), extrinsic (dependent on the intervention or guidance of an outside person or medium), or a combination of the two.
9. Whether there are any specific recommendations for type or control of breathing, or whether a normal breathing pattern is to be maintained. …

(Nash and Newberg, 2023)

This classification system offers the most comprehensive approach out of those I have seen and if classifications might be a way that you find it helpful to understand and categorise practices generally, then I'd encourage you to refer back to it when approaching the different MMs in this book. However, I will be utilising the meditation framework as already presented. Given that this suitable classification already exists it could seem that I am unnecessarily reinventing the wheel. However, I think as I am firstly describing a specific mindset from various psychotherapy modalities, so taking a more phenomenological perspective and then matching a meditation technique to that, I have found a more phenomenological framework to fit better with the task in hand. However, the above classifications that take a phenomenological approach seem either so simple they are exclusionary, or incorporating everything, but too complex to be useful. I have also developed this framework specifically to be used alongside psychotherapy approaches. This framework also has a more practical function as opposed to the more academic nature of a classification system and is very much focussed on outcomes. This allows the descriptions of mindsets to be mapped onto the framework and a MM extrapolated from that. These processes that are embedded in the meditation instructions match tier 3 of the Nash and Newberg classification.

In his excellent book, *Mindfulness Meditation in Psychotherapy; An Integrated Model for Clinicians*, Steven Alper (2016) presents a mindfulness pyramid: An integrated model of mindfulness to help understand mindfulness meditation as it relates to psychotherapy. This is probably the most similar publication to this book in its focus solely on how meditation can enhance a psychotherapist's approach, albeit coming from a different angle by applying the mindfulness pyramid to the common factors of all psychotherapists. I find this pyramid to be comprehensive for the purpose of portraying the different aspects of mindfulness in this general way:

> I describe this model as "transtheoretical" because it's based on the assumption that mindfulness, whether or not it's labeled as such, undergirds and informs all effective psychotherapy regardless of theory or technique.
>
> (Alper, 2016, p. 35)

However, unlike this and other books written on the topic (McCollum, 2014; Siegel, 2010), I am coming from the perspective that each of the described psychotherapy models has different mindsets and therefore require specific MMs to engender these frames of mind. Therefore, while this model suits Alper's aims, I feel that the framework below offers a more specific approach for the focus of this book, which I hope will become more apparent in the rest of this chapter and beyond. My definition of meditation that began the chapter is also very simple – broad enough to incorporate all the techniques described in the book but acknowledging the unique nature of meditation without it simply becoming anything whereby you might be in a focussed state of mind.

What Meditation Is Not

I think it is helpful at this early stage having established a framework around what meditation is, to bring in some commonly held misconceptions and discuss what falls outside of the boundaries of meditation. First, it is not the aim of meditation to be not thinking in order to reach some sort of blank mindset. Perhaps a particularly quiet state of mind might arise as a result of a very concentrated mind, but as will be explored later and also in the *Troubleshooting* section, if one puts that as the aim, then it will inevitably result in lots of thinking and agitation. Many people I teach meditation to tell me that they can't meditate because when they sit down to begin, they are thinking too much. It is often a relief for them to hear that not thinking isn't the aim but is often the result of a persistent practice. In many meditation traditions, there is also a big focus on staying in the present moment as a goal of meditation. This is rightly so, but I prefer to come from it at a slightly different angle that can loosen things up if it is a struggle to maintain that present moment perspective. We have already thought about mindfulness and ardency as using the past and future as a function of meditation technique. I also want to emphasise that being present is not the end point of the meditation but rather the beginning. That it is once we are dwelling in the present that we can *do* something there. That could be something active like a visualisation or a body scan, but equally might be about allowing an experience to unfold. Either way, the present moment isn't the goal but a platform or stage from which the meditation practice can take place.

Linked to this concept, there can also be a focus on reaching some kind of trance-like state. I think of a trance-like state as incorporating both a state of mindlessness and euphoria. While it might seem like quite a pleasant state, I'm not sure it is one that is conducive to the outcomes described above of concentration or discernment but is more like a kind of seemingly pleasant but unengaged state of mind. That may be desirable for people who are aiming for pleasant states or have a certain belief that this means there is some sort of communing with a divine being, but it is not of concern for our purposes here. As for other unusual experiences, such as hallucinations or extra corporeal phenomena that can arise from meditation, this may occur and it is best to consult with a meditation teacher to think together about the meaning of them and how they might connect to practice. However, again, these experiences are not the focus of the sorts of meditation as defined in this book.

When discussing meditation informally with others, they will tell me that going for a run, some other kind of exercise, or artistic activity is their meditation. I think while they might be relaxing activities and people may be in a state of flow while doing them, I wouldn't classify it as meditation simply for the fact that the aim and focus of the main activity is something else, such as sport or physical fitness and a relaxing state comes as a byproduct. In meditation, it is the state of awareness, the specific kind of attention which forms the content of the activity rather than a process of relaxation or flow being mediated through another activity. Meditation is ultimately engaged with getting into contact with our own awareness and sensory phenomena in as direct and unmediated manner as one can reach with the focus of developing concentration and discernment.

While relaxation may very well be an outcome of meditation, it is not always so. Sometimes, challenging and uncomfortable states may arise. This doesn't mean a practitioner is doing something wrong, but that when training the mind in a different way of being, you can come up against a whole variety of resistances and discomforts both mental and physical. That said, overall, I usually advise people that the general trend of a committed meditation practice should be a calmer and kinder outlook with reference to themselves, others and their environment.

It is also necessary to explain that meditation does not necessarily equate to a pleasant experience or any of the more mystical experiences that you might have heard from many of the spiritual traditions involving euphoric or blissful states. That said, they might arise in your practice, but this shouldn't be the focus and as with not thinking, if it is, they wouldn't arise anyway. Due to much of the imagery around meditation showing either a monk in robes or some kind of model sitting with a knowing smile, in a beautiful environment, there can be an ingrained cultural expectation to have that sort of experience.

On the other side of the coin, another misconception and driver for beginners to give up is coming up against mental or physical discomfort. I remember as a child being fascinated by the page in my encyclopaedia on Buddhism – trying to follow the meditation instructions in a small box on the side of the page, but finding the psychological discomfort too much after a short period of time and stopping. It took many years before I was drawn back to practise. Just as therapy can often be a bumpy ride, so meditation can be physically and emotionally uncomfortable. The troubleshooting chapter will go someway to support you to mitigate these discomforts, however, they are inescapable.

Be it the absence of very blissful states or being exposed to lots of pain, one can be left very critical of meditation as a harmful and unpleasant experience. When I took one of my first intensive silent meditation retreats in India after my medical elective around twelve years ago, I was sharing a room with a young Australian yoga enthusiast. For the whole retreat, I was incredibly uncomfortable sitting on the floor in the scorching Indian summer heat trying my best to arrange cushions to alleviate myself of my soreness, much of which, as I eventually discovered was more a physical manifestation of psychological discomfort than my lack of flexibility. Meanwhile, my roommate was sitting with perfect posture throughout and I imagined him in some kind of deep concentration or blissful state. When we were finally able to talk at the end of the retreat, he let me know that appearances can be deceptive, and he was in great mental and physical discomfort for much of the beginning of the retreat as I was. Not too long after that, I took another similar meditation retreat and sat with far less discomfort and far more moments of peace and insight. It was not that I had suddenly become more flexible and able to sit on the floor in comfort, but I had trained my mind to be far less restless, which resulted in a very different experience. So, there may very well be pain, but also, we can adapt, change, manage it and become more robust and resilient through meditation, and also have experiences of deep peace, insight and calm.

Psychotherapy and Meditation in Theory and Practice

Technique and practice, while important in both psychotherapy and meditation do differ. Practice in psychotherapy is broadly within the confines of a relationship between two people, but meditation forms a more individual reflective experience albeit often with external guidance, analogous to the relationship of a therapist and supervisor. In meditation, the relationship is between different parts of the mind with a more external guiding and interactive learning environment outside of this (be that this book, a teacher or fellow meditators). In psychotherapy, there are also ongoing processes occurring within the client's mind and their unconscious as much as with the therapist. It is the external setting and the therapist's internal setting that helps to facilitate this, which acts more directly than a guide to a meditator. However, this is more influenced by the therapist than the client themselves. For both, the development of the practice is an iterative process of positive feedback, one where technique is constantly being revised and returned to, albeit without an idea of perfecting said technique and then stopping. Instead, it is a process essential to the development of the practice in and of itself.

In terms of technique, meditation describes specific ways of interacting with the self and then consequentially another. Psychotherapy also establishes this, but the other way around, through the relationship between therapist and client creating that change within the self for the client. In both meditation and psychotherapy, techniques are not generalisable to everyone and must adapt to the specific person. In this way, both methods require a teacher or guide with more experience to guide the subject in a bespoke manner towards the required outcome.

Both meditation and psychotherapy have a great diversity in technique and can differ hugely between traditions. Both also rely on the development of an attitude which is broadly consistent between traditions. For example, all therapists will be active listeners and empathic, which is explored more in the section on *A General Therapeutic Stance*. In all meditation techniques, concentration and discernment are embedded. It is the nature of these attitudes through technique, informed by theory, which differs.

There are also other similarities between meditation and psychotherapy traditions. Already mentioned would be the concept of an internal setting, a description of the mindset established and developed in both trainings. Self-awareness is of course, crucial for a therapist to prevent the therapist breaking boundaries or reacting with action to something that might be perceived as a provocation from a client. In meditation, self-awareness naturally arises through the process of paying attention and, therefore, observing what's occurring in the mind and body. An already mentioned typical experience for a beginner meditator might be noticing just how much the mind bounces about from thought to thought and sensation to sensation, which, while it might be known anyway, is truly experienced in its most full and often uncomfortable way when sitting down and occupying a position of observation. Sometimes felt to be a failure for a beginner, but noticing that the mind is bubbling away like this is an important step towards greater self-awareness. Becoming aware of this, beginning to tolerate it and hopefully finding that by not reacting, it begins to settle down is a big achievement. Repeating this process, learning how to use the meditation object to settle the mind and increase focus can bring about a reduction of ruminations, but more as a side effect than an aim itself. At the same time, it can very often be too big an obstacle for a beginner preventing continuation on the very brink of an important insight.

When faced with the whole range of emotions that a client brings to the consulting room, robustness is another important feature in psychotherapy and is shared with meditation. Robustness or resilience helps to keep the therapist level-headed when they might be faced with high levels of distress. It is especially the aspect of mindfulness, remembering to keep the meditation object in mind which helps to develop this faculty. Every time the mind wanders from the meditation object, the mind remembers it is trying to focus on the object and attention is brought back in an empathic way. This action, when faced with a range of physical and psychological experiences in meditation that might urge the meditator to stop altogether, helps to develop this capacity and is necessary as one of the factors which can be the focus of ardency – to take up in the future through practice. Just as with psychotherapy, it is important not to see this as the primary focus; too much robustness makes us impervious and cold. It is crucial to have that balance to remain sensitive enough without being swept away. Bringing in empathy towards ourselves when practising helps to modify some of the discomfort and potential frustration, also balancing this potential for detachment. There are also ways to meditate, which bring about more pleasant sensations which can make a more focussed state of mind more desirable than the temptations of mind wandering, daydreaming and fantasising.

Lastly, the importance of establishing a frame is present for both. In psychotherapy, this is generally thought of as a reasonably consistent environment, including the location and timing, but also other aspects comprising confidentiality, reliability of the therapist and the emotional environment, which inevitably derives from the therapist's internal setting. The establishment of the meditation frame will be explored in the first guided meditation at the end of the chapter encompassing location, timing, physical position and regularity. Just as in psychotherapy, this is established at each session functioning to ground the mind in the body and creating a modicum of calm.

What About Mindfulness?

First, I think it is helpful to note the origins of the use of the word mindfulness as a descriptor for a certain aspect of meditation as I have used it, or for the whole meditation itself as is common in recent years. The British translator of Buddhist texts, Thomas Rhys Davids, who founded the Pāli Text society in 1881 (Pāli being the language of the earliest Buddhist texts) selected it as the translation of the word sati (Alabaster, 1871, p.197) beating him to the use of the word with a translation of sati as *the act of keeping oneself mindful*). Sati is present in descriptions of meditation practice as well as one of the factors in the eight-fold noble path in Buddhism, which is a guide to the way out of stress and suffering. Rhy Davids most probably adapted the word mindful from the Anglican prayer before meals, changing it from the adjective mindful to the noun mindfulness:

> *Give us grateful hearts,*
> *O Father, for all thy mercies,*
> *And make us mindful*
> *Of the needs of others;*
> *Through Jesus Christ our Lord.*
> *Amen.*

The etymology of the word sati itself points towards a description that is closer to *remembering to observe*, joining aspects of remembering and observing together. Therefore, the English word mindfulness is already an approximation of the original meaning of the word (Walpola, Walpola and Toneatto, 2022), but the aspect of remembering is a central part of it. Some contemporary languages also point towards this, such as Javanese, spoken by people from Java, Indonesia. Javanese has etymological origins in Sanskrit that is consequentially derived from Pali. In Javanese the word for remember – *eling* is the same as the word for mindful.

In addition, it might come as a surprise that in Buddhism, the religion probably most associated with meditation and the techniques from which have formed many secular mindfulness practices, there isn't actually a specific word for meditation in the early texts. Practitioners were instead urged to concentrate their minds or develop mindfulness to establish certain mental states of high concentration or insights into the nature of reality. Sometimes, the word bhāvanā in Pali, roughly translated as becoming or development, padhāna meaning striving, and others can be thought of as analogous to meditation. Therefore, the word mindfulness has filled some of this gap.

The contemporary psychological mindfulness movement defines mindfulness as

> … the awareness that emerges through paying attention on purpose, in the present moment and nonjudgmentally, to things as they are.
>
> (Segal, Williams and Teasdale, 2013, p. 132)

This is from its probably the most well-known application in therapy for mindfulness-based cognitive behaviour therapy (MBCT) and also mindfulness-based stress reduction (MBSR) (Kabat-Zinn, 2013). Using the meditation framework above, this could be defined as a more open, non-judgemental awareness where alertness to the present moment is most emphasised.

In MBSR and MBCT mindfulness *is* meditation. In contrast, I have presented mindfulness simply as remembering to keep an object in mind, which is a more specific, narrow definition, similar to the early Buddhist meaning of sati above, where sati was but one aspect of a description of a practice that incorporated different features, not just remembering to keep the object in mind. Therefore, by putting mindfulness into a larger stable with other mental qualities, each mental quality can be investigated and adjusted to bring about different outcomes. This means meditation techniques can be tailored to those mental qualities that a specific internal therapeutic setting may require. The contemporary mindfulness definition as a complete meditation technique would not allow for any changes with only a present moment, open, non-judgemental type of awareness utilised. While this mindset could be applied to different meditation objects such as the breath, while walking or specific body parts, the present moment, open, non-judgemental perspective remains constant. So, for example, as more thoroughly explained later, at times it can be advantageous to alter the meditation object, such as the breath, rather than accept, however, it may be at the time, taking a less non-judgemental and more discerning attitude. Therefore, while mindfulness by this definition has its place and purpose, it couldn't be altered and adapted as I am working towards in this book and, therefore, has not been used, despite perhaps being a more familiar approach.

That's not to say that the above technique is intrinsically less helpful than others. All practitioners of MBSR, MBCT and the other therapies that incorporate mindfulness into their treatment are encouraged to maintain their own practice, just as many psychotherapists will often maintain their own treatment with a therapist generally from their own modality. With MBCT practitioners, maintaining a mindfulness practice is both to inform their work as therapists but more so for them to get the benefits of the mindfulness work themselves. Of course, there is a huge body of evidence that shows how this technique in concert with different therapeutic approaches has a huge potential to support people.

What I would say, is I find this style of mindfulness meditation can be quite a challenging technique with which to begin practising meditation. By employing open awareness combined with a non-judgemental approach, a meditator has to contend with quite a lot of raw experiences coming into the mind due to this choiceless attention, which can be overwhelming to someone who may not yet have the mental strength to manage such unfiltered thoughts, feelings and emotions arising. Once mental robustness has been developed, or perhaps is already present, this style of meditation is incredibly powerful. I have found that this approach of choiceless awareness can bring about a great sense of ease and calm when I have already reached a place that can tolerate its various challenges, after say using the breath or another object to alter and calm various emotional, physical and physical experiences.

There has been a move towards incorporating a wider range of techniques taught into mindfulness teacher training and delivery in the past ten years for this reason, of which this book forms a part. A study of 64 randomly selected therapists in German found that while 82% reported using mindfulness techniques sometimes with their clients, most offer that in a more eclectic manner than is described by their trainings (Michalak, Steinhaus and Heidenreich, 2018). Therefore, there is a desire to seek out methods beyond these most well-known approaches. That said, this technique is most often thought of as associated with the word mindfulness, or what is sometimes referred to as *mindfulness meditation*. I have continued to use the word as I think it sums up the definition I am using well. I hope these paragraphs have served to clear up any confusion.

Responding to Criticisms

There are a host of criticisms about meditation of which the reader may be aware, which I think would be helpful to acknowledge both in order to recognise the limitations of meditation, and also address and counter some of the others. I will try to show how they might relate to the use of meditation for psychotherapists and some of the ways in which this book manages them. It is important to recognise that psychotherapy, as practised in most contexts, has been dominated by thinking and research from a Western and predominately Eurocentric perspective. Bringing in cultural practices from outside is I believe, an enriching process. However, it can be experienced as an intrusion especially when these might originate from religions borne from thousands of years of anecdotal experience rather than an empirically tested science. I think this has decreased in recent years, given the amount of research around mindfulness and the engagement of traditions such as Tibetan Buddhism with neuroscience (Davidson and Lutz, 2008). However, we can see how external influences have been rejected in psychotherapy starting from the early days of psychoanalysis.

Criticism of meditation in relation to psychotherapy can be tracked back to the 1930s. In Civilisation and its Discontents, Sigmund Freud, the Austrian neurologist and founder of psychoanalysis (1930, p. 79), describes ... *wordly wisdom from the East* in a sarcastic manner when discussing the issue of religion and the oceanic feeling which was brought to his attention in correspondence with the French Nobel winning novelist and essayist Romain Rolland. This oceanic feeling, inspired by the Indian mystic Ramakrishna, equated to a spiritual or religious feeling of oneness with the universe characterised by deep levels of concentration or samadhi as it is known in the Sanskrit of Hinduism or Pali of Buddhism.

Broadly speaking, this oceanic feeling can also be found in other meditation traditions. The Vipassana-ñāṇas (Mahasi, 2016) are signposts of comprehension reached as levels of insight into the nature of reality. In early Buddhism, the jhānas, different levels of mental absorption that can be used to shine a light on reality, are defined by the degree of samadhi or right concentration in the eight-fold noble path, which is the road map to Nibbana or enlightenment. In Zen Buddhism moments of satori, realising one's nature, can come from moments of deep meditation or no mind practice. All three examples can be characterised by some feelings akin to this oceanic feeling, the trance-like states I wrote of before and are also present in the Abrahamic traditions in a range of practices, including Christian monastic chanting, Sufi whirling dervishes dancing and Jewish Hasidic devekut niggunim prayers. We will speak more about some of these experiences as understood through a neuroscientific lens later and when thinking about what is known as the subtle body.

Freud's dispute with this oceanic feeling seems to rest on a practice which indeed is antithetical to most therapeutic approaches and the evenly suspended attention which he proposed. Freud suggests that these states are used to avoid discomfort by *killing off the instincts* (Freud, 1930, p. 79). Freud compares this with a narcissistic type of person who instead of seeking pleasure, avoids suffering and goes on to suggest that *if it succeeds, then the subject has, it is true, given up all other activities as well – he has sacrificed his life*. This mindset would, of course, be antithetical to the therapist, who must engage with discomfort to make sense of it rather than repress or act on it.

In addition, I agree that this level of absorption and concentration is not necessarily helpful for a therapist given the attention needed to focus on the client too. I think in the popular imagination, meditation is often thought of in this way. Perhaps when thinking of a meditative state, an image of a monk or nun in a blissful state of deep concentration is conjured up, with them either floating in the air or with a bright light shining above their head as an optional addition. The truth is that monastics can struggle with their meditation practice as much as a lay person, if not more due to their commitment to practice, and that while these blissful states can arise, much of the work can be challenging and painful. Work is also done *off the cushion* when integrating meditation and the lessons from it into everyday life just as this book proposes.

The framework and techniques described in this book seek to show how meditation techniques can be adapted so that these oceanic feelings or deep states of concentration do not interfere, but rather an appropriate level of concentration and a particular internal setting is reached, which is more in line with the psychotherapy modalities described. As will be shown, focus and concentration are required, but at a specific level whereby that focus can then be used in the room with a client or to become more self-aware. There needs to be a balance with receptiveness so that the therapist is not totally impervious to the client's experience. I think the idea of a therapist as some kind of impenetrable mirror delivering wisdom to a client from on high is now, fortunately an idea of a more historical and paternalistic model. Rather, the therapist is in the midst of an emotional experience with the client so must be sensitive albeit robust, focussed but also receptive and maintaining an empathic and resilient presence. Meditation using my proposed techniques can help achieve this balance, hopefully avoiding the pitfall of being lost in some kind of oceanic feeling or becoming too disengaged and detached from the impact of others.

Aside from the discussion about the secular mindfulness approach, other literature has also focussed on wider social issues and how a purely non-judgement, accepting and open awareness can lead to meditators becoming too accommodating of environments which might actually be harmful. This has been expressed in a workplace situation, especially those in a more corporate environment, where mindfulness has been pushed by executives to allow unhealthy work environments to be tolerated by their workers that would otherwise be deemed unacceptable. This concept can then be extended throughout society as a kind of mindlessness, whereby citizens accept whatever situation is thrown at them without taking on any external social or political activism, the responsibility for difficulties and also the solution to those being shifted entirely onto the individual (Purser, 2019). I have a lot of sympathy for this position and don't necessarily think teaching certain meditations is helpful everywhere. For this reason, it might be more supportive to teach a meditation technique which is more discerning and focussed, allowing a meditator to develop these capacities in other areas of their lives.

I also don't think a mindfulness course would intentionally teach this, but having spoken to many people exposed to this secular mindfulness approach, it can be unknowingly taken in. As mentioned above, by initially making judgements and choices in meditation, one can reach a place where this non-judgemental practice might be more appropriate and the meditator is more able to notice when the mind makes certain decisions and change them, rather than operating in a more accepting mode. A meditation practice that isn't entirely choiceless can bring these more unconscious decision processes into the light of day. The development of so-called second-generation mindfulness-based interventions takes this issue into account, including both more active and evaluating or discriminative forms of meditative awareness within a more overtly spiritual infrastructure (Shonin and Van Gordon, 2014; Van Gordon, Shonin and Griffiths, 2015).

There is also the issue of morality and ethics. An entirely secular approach removes these aspects, which are a central part of spiritual development in the faiths from which many of these approaches derive. There is an appropriation of but one section of the practice or faith – meditation and a rejection of those ethical aspects. Sometimes, I get the sense that there is a view in secular meditation that such issues are unnecessary, condescending, archaic and personally intrusive. At the same time, insisting on certain morals or virtues has a distinctive paternalistic and historically almost Victorian attitude. I would argue that a firm footing in ethics is a prerequisite for working as a therapist as it grounds clinicians in concepts of compassion towards ourselves and others and respect for others and the environment. This in turn, leads to confidence for the therapist to be able to work with clients and, therefore, for the client to be able to trust the therapist sufficiently. Likewise, I think it is supportive for a meditation practice by keeping certain harmful behaviours towards the self and others at bay, which can increase mental distress, but also for the same reasons as why it is essential for working as a therapist. This might bring us to more of an attitude of integrity and probity rather than a potentially meaningless and alienating list of requirements. A strong set of ethical guidelines and boundaries, therefore not only creates a stable frame for therapy to occur, but also the environment for a more steady mindset from which the therapeutic relationship can emerge. For the same reasons, this level headedness also creates a firm foundation for meditation practice.

Therefore, prohibitions of potentially harmful behaviours aren't necessarily coming from the position of a belief in a faith or holy book but can include that which all therapists subscribe to by virtue of their registration to a regulatory body. All regulatory bodies will have not only a code of ethics, which a therapist keeps to, but also processes by which clients can make complaints if their therapist falls short. I think that this could be viewed as equivalent to a set of morals or ethics by which people of faith follow and offers a similar grounding for meditation practice as outlined above. At the same time, they are an understandable and palatable form of an approach that develops integrity. Therefore, just as a psychotherapist who might take alcohol socially would never consider this when working with clients, I would expect them to refrain when meditating. However, to be clear I will not be making any demands of readers about their behaviour and the only expectations will be around curiosity and a certain amount of open-mindedness to giving a fair trial to the ideas and practices proposed.

Meditation is still a relatively new approach to many, especially in therapy circles, which means some will be very enthusiastic about its potential. I think that when any new approach is established, there can be such a desire to show its benefits that it can sometimes be offered as a panacea. A backlash can then grow with some of those criticisms towards meditation being addressed here. It is important to acknowledge that meditation may not be appropriate everywhere and its limitations have been seen in studies. For example, one of the largest studies into the effectiveness of mindfulness was undertaken to look at the impact of mindfulness on students at school. The randomised controlled trial involved 84 schools and 8,376 pupils, but did not find the positive outcome for pupils as expected (Montero-Marin et al., 2022) and I would hope that, therefore, the use of mindfulness for students at schools might have to be reviewed. Due to the risks of generalisability, I have purposefully shown how meditation can be connected to specific therapy modalities rather than produce a general book on the benefits of different techniques for all therapists, and why I make sure to emphasise that meditation is an adjunct rather than a replacement to different training methods.

In terms of the dangers of meditation, they have been documented thoroughly (Farias et al., 2020; Goldberg et al., 2022; Goyal et al., 2014) with depression, anxiety, dissociation and even psychotic events described. A causal relationship is not always so clear, incidence varies depending on criteria and it hasn't always been found that a meditator wasn't glad to have tried it depending on the amount of distress that was experienced.

There is also evidence that the level of meditation experience is not necessarily linked to reducing adverse events so even if someone has been meditating for a long time, there is potential for them to experience difficulties. It has also been found that mental distress might be more common than somatic discomfort and that face-to-face delivery of meditation teaching can increase these risks. It is important to note that the meditation might also not be causing these adverse events but is making participants more conscious of experiences that may have been out of their awareness until they begin meditating (Taylor et al., 2022). Therefore, it is important to be aware of potential pitfalls in practising meditation as well as having others on hand for support, conscious of what might be challenging for people learning meditation. I have witnessed high levels of mental distress at meditation retreats, which can be intense by virtue of the amount of time meditating due to retreats often held in near complete silence and sometimes staff working there not being trained in how to work with people in high levels of mental distress. When it comes to the population whom this book is directed at, namely psychotherapists qualified and in training as well as others working in a range of professions supporting those experiencing mental distress, I am not of the belief that meditation is particularly dangerous unless approached either especially intensely like on one of those retreats and if the person is in a fragile mental state.

This idea that many of the negative reactions from meditation represent issues that are already present, but the effect of meditating exposes them when defence mechanisms are reduced can be thought of as similar to when starting therapy. The start of therapeutic work might end up stirring up more anxiety for a client in these initial stages. Therefore, if you do experience any very strong physical, emotional or psychological reaction, then it would be best to approach a medical professional or psychotherapist as appropriate. For the same reason, a gradual approach to training in meditation is advisable, steadily building up the length and frequency of sessions, reviewing and addressing any difficulties or challenging experiences along the way. It might make sense to spend a lot of time on the initial meditation exercise of establishing the meditation frame and the exploration of the breath in order to have a firm foundation for the rest of the practices. There is plenty in the meditation instructions and the latter chapters to provide a range of practices and responses to difficulties that might suit different people before going towards the more in-depth and complex techniques that are presented as associated with specific therapeutic approaches. Working on meditation with other people also offers a stronger structure for collaborative work, management of potential anxieties that emerge and the sharing of techniques to work with different challenges.

I have also heard of meditation being accused as a kind of unnecessary navel-gazing which promotes a narcissistic focus on the self. That said, I have heard the same about psychotherapy from people bemoaning how society has become self-obsessed and that therapy promotes a self-centred blame culture. I'll leave this attitude towards psychotherapy to one side as I expect most readers will be familiar with the various responses. With regards to meditation, they probably run along similar lines. The one that might resonate most with the expected audience of this book is that by meditating and developing the various different benefits, it places you at a much better place to enhance your therapeutic practice and support others. I have also avoided practices in this book that promote the highest levels of concentration and mental absorption, whereby there is a focus on pleasant bodily sensations and certain hallucinations, which, in my mind, are not related to the aims of this book. It is probably these methods which those people who make these accusations are thinking of when they talk down meditation as a possible route towards improving the quality of interpersonal relationships.

The Current Evidence Base

There have been a variety of studies, mostly over the last twenty years, which investigate the benefits of meditation for psychotherapists and psychologists practising therapy especially those in training. It should be noted that none of them are particularly large scale and there is a wide diversity in the meditation techniques employed, sometimes based on Zen Buddhism, an MBSR course or more towards developing compassion. Nonetheless, I think as a body of evidence, these studies offer supporting data to promote a wider uptake of meditation by psychotherapists, but in a more structured way. I think it also provides a rationale for incorporating some meditation teaching within therapy trainings beyond those whereby mindfulness is part of the treatment itself.

Mindfulness training for all healthcare professionals has been established as reducing distress and improving wellbeing, but then that is known to be the case for the general population, too, so it is unsurprising (Spinelli, Wisener and Khoury, 2019). I have found the same from my own experience of teaching health and social care students, their feedback let me know how useful it is to have methods they can rely on to manage stressful work situations. However, the remit of this book is beyond stress management. What follows is a survey of studies specifically involving psychotherapists based on the benefits examined. Anecdotally, I have heard therapists describe how they wished that there was a technique that would allow them to become more robust, or more in touch with the mindset that they might be aiming to develop. Often, the finger is pointed towards having more personal therapy, supervision or seminars. I think meditation offers a refreshing alternative which is empowering due to the ability to practise alone as well as in groups, is inexpensive to deliver and doesn't require any special equipment or location. Many therapists are already practising a range of meditation techniques, often the ones which they also use therapeutically with clients, but also those associated with spiritual development and sometimes religious beliefs too (Michalak et al., 2018). However, these practices often fall short of those recommended to clients, most like for a variety of reasons that will be explored in the *Troubleshooting* chapter later in this book. Many therapists will already be practising meditation independently and most likely will have made many of the connections I will write about in this book. I think by attaching meditation practice to professional as well as personal development it adds more impetus to the development of a meaningful habit.

Looking from the perspective of the therapist, one systematic review of the literature found that when mindfulness-based interventions are applied to psychotherapists, they report a limited increase in their own empathy (Garrote-Caparrós et al., 2021) rather than an effect on the therapeutic alliance or on clients' symptoms. While therapists might find improvements in their own clinical capabilities, this isn't always reflected in the evidence from a client's perspective (Swift et al., 2017). There is also some evidence that while the client's symptoms might not decrease, there is significant patient-rated improvements in interpersonal functioning (Ryan et al., 2012).

The emphasis on increased therapist empathy, as well as mindfulness, has been repeated elsewhere when using an MBCT course for trainee clinical psychologists (Hopkins and Proeve, 2013) and with a similar method and cohort finding increased empathy and mindfulness alongside self-compassion and less rumination (Rimes and Wingrove, 2010). So, this puts the emphasis on the effect of the meditation on the therapist's experience rather than the clinical outcome which might seem a bit counter intuitive as if it isn't affecting the client outcome, then the purpose might seem limited. First, empathy being one of the common factors between all therapeutic modalities, as illustrated in more depth in the section on *A General Therapeutic Stance*, makes it a very desirable outcome. Also, measurements of clinical outcomes in therapeutic studies don't always give the full picture due to changes that may occur beyond the study's length. When judging success by a reduction in client symptoms, there is the challenge that these change over time, and there could be a time-delayed effect on improvement after a piece of therapy work whereby loss of the therapy and the therapist causes a brief return of symptoms before independence returns and the results of the therapy are really felt. There is also the challenge of fitting a qualitative experience into quantitative data, which runs across all studies involving psychotherapy. This can be countered by running larger randomised controlled studies. The field of research into therapy and meditation thought has not reached the point at which these studies are deemed desirable enough to be undertaken. However, as shown below other studies do find positive clinical outcomes, so it is a mixed picture. Other studies have shown that delivering a general programme specifically for therapists can deliver a more balanced and accepting attitude for the therapist (Aggs and Bambling, 2010), especially in accepting without judgement (Kalmar et al., 2024) supporting the development of a range of aspects of the therapeutic internal setting.

From the client's perspective, when promoting mindfulness in psychotherapists who are in training, it can influence the treatment results positively for clients (Grepmair et al., 2007a; Grepmair et al., 2007b). Even if clients don't feel the therapist is more present, they find the sessions more effective with therapists who have had some meditation training (Ivanovic et al., 2015). Clients can experience the therapist as more empathic with a reflected therapist-client bond and consequentially improved symptoms (Garrote-Caparrós et al., 2022). As the relationship between therapist and client is the most positive indicator for success of therapy this is a highly desirable outcome and one which seems to be rooted in an increase in empathy from the therapist. I also expect the general reduction in anxiety and increased presence of the therapist is picked up by clients and can be a possible mechanism by which meditation can enhance clinical practice especially in therapists who are currently training where anxiety levels might be higher than those therapists with more experience.

In terms of resilience and robustness, it has been found that trainees can experience an increase in attention and the capacity to manage anger after an eight-week mindfulness training (Rodriguez Vega et al., 2013). Likewise, therapeutic presence, attention and empathy is found to increase (Keane, 2013) as well as self-compassion (Bourgault and Dionne, 2018). This suggests an increase in robustness that can occur through the practice translates into the ability for therapists to manage their own emotions. In the context of countertransference, it has been shown that therapists can increase awareness of their own countertransference with a more objective observational stance and enable a more compassionate and curious stance (Millon and Halewood, 2015). It appears that the length of time of meditation experience over years is more important than a short-term effect in the management of countertransference offering support for the idea of integrating meditation into a training experience (Fatter and Hayes, 2013).

Meditation also can help to develop an increase in self-care by taking on a compassion-based mindfulness practice, again with length of practice emphasised (Christopher et al., 2010; Hunt et al., 2021) and reduce the risk of compassion fatigue (Dorian and Killebrew, 2014), one of the markers on the way to burnout. This capacity can be developed not just through the process of compassion but also by therapists generally reducing stress (Felton, Coates and Christopher, 2013; Shapiro, Brown and Biegel, 2007) or through a general mindfulness practice which engenders self-compassion as well as towards others through modifying their reactions to life experiences in a less reactive way (Lalor and Khoshfetrat, 2023; Latorre et al., 2021) which of course can lead to being a more effective therapist who is more resilient to the pressures of being around and taking on so much mental distress and the chance of vicarious traumatisation.

I think as this is a relatively niche area of research, most studies have aimed at showing a change in the therapist's experience as, in a way, it is them undergoing the intervention. It has yet to be established about how best a training might work or what kind of meditation might be most effective. It has been found that a shorter format of practice with clinical psychology trainees was effective in producing many of the effects described above in terms of personal and professional development (Hemanth and Fisher, 2014), even utilising ten minutes during lunch breaks for other trainee clinical psychologists (Moore, 2008) showing that an integration of this teaching doesn't necessarily need to come at the expense of other established training methods. In terms of when to practice meditation so as to benefit most from the fruits of practice, one study looked at using a centring technique five minutes before a session with therapists feeling more single minded. Although clients didn't notice this, they did find the session more effective (Dunn et al., 2013). In the penultimate chapter of the book looking at *Other Complementary Techniques* that might not fit in with specific therapy modalities, I make suggestions of MMs that you can utilise before, during and after a session.

A focus of future studies will be to see if there is a significant impact for clients after speaking with a therapist who has developed a robust practice beyond a brief training in meditation on top of their standard therapeutic training. There is also definitely space for a study, over a longer period of time involving comparing whole cohorts of therapists in the same trainings either receiving meditation training or having the standard training for that course. This could assess changes from both the therapist and clients' perspectives and could provide some more robust evidence to support the hypothesis of this book. While I know that for me and other clinicians I have spoken with who practise meditation have found it to be hugely beneficial for our clinical practice, the current evidence base is not so strong. There have been so many preliminary studies as outlined above, and I would be keen to progress with this idea at a training institute that might be interested in taking up meditation as a formal training technique alongside already established methods. I think this would make more or a case for the wider practice of meditation in the psychotherapy profession.

Chapter Summary

- ◆ The meditation framework allows different types of practices to be defined by how they develop different kinds of concentration (open or focussed) and discernment (evaluating or non-judgemental)
- ◆ MMs can focus more on different aspects of mindfulness, alertness and ardency, each representing aspects of the time continuum – past, present and future, respectively
- ◆ There are a multitude of different classifications already developed around meditation, each with its own perspectives, the meditation framework has been developed more for the purposes of this book
- ◆ Meditation has a number of misconceptions around it as well as criticisms, some based on these misapprehensions, others due to an understanding around a more limited view of what meditation might entail

- ◆ While the practice of meditation and psychotherapy have many similarities, there are also differences
- ◆ Secular mindfulness, while very important in its clinical application, also has some limitations
- ◆ There is a body of evidence for using meditation to enhance the clinical skills of a psychotherapist, which are mostly based on common factors for all therapies and more general MMs.

References

Aggs, C. and Bambling, M. (2010). Teaching mindfulness to psychotherapists in clinical practice: The mindful therapy programme. *Counselling and Psychotherapy Research*, 10(4), pp.278–286.

Alabaster, H. (1871). *The Wheel of the Law. Buddhism Illustrated from Siamese Sources*. London: Trübner.

Alper, S.A. (2016). *Mindfulness Meditation in Psychotherapy*. California, CA: New Harbinger Publications.

Bourgault, M. and Dionne, F. (2018). Therapeutic presence and mindfulness: Mediating role of self-compassion and psychological distress among psychologists. *Mindfulness*, 10(4), pp.650–656.

Christopher, J.C., Chrisman, J.A., Trotter-Mathison, M.J., Schure, M.B., Dahlen, P. and Christopher, S.B. (2010). Perceptions of the long-term influence of mindfulness training on counselors and psychotherapists. *Journal of Humanistic Psychology*, 51(3), pp.318–349.

Davidson, R.J. and Lutz, A. (2008). Buddha's brain: Neuroplasticity and meditation. *IEEE Signal Processing Magazine*, 25(1), pp.176–174.

Dorian, M. and Killebrew, J.E. (2014). A study of mindfulness and self-care: A path to self-compassion for female therapists in training. *Women & Therapy*, 37(1–2), pp.155–163.

Dunn, R., Callahan, J.L., Swift, J.K. and Ivanovic, M. (2013). Effects of pre-session centering for therapists on session presence and effectiveness. *Psychotherapy Research*, 23(1), pp.78–85.

Engström, M., Willander, J. and Simon, R. (2021). A review of the methodology, taxonomy, and definitions in recent fMRI research on meditation. *Mindfulness*, 13(3), pp.541–555.

Farias, M., Maraldi, E., Wallenkampf, K.C. and Lucchetti, G. (2020). Adverse events in meditation practices and meditation-based therapies: A systematic review. *Acta Psychiatrica Scandinavica*, 142(5), pp.374–393.

Fatter, D.M. and Hayes, J.A. (2013). What facilitates countertransference management? The roles of therapist meditation, mindfulness, and self-differentiation. *Psychotherapy Research*, 23(5), pp.502–513.

Felton, T.M., Coates, L. and Christopher, J.C. (2013). Impact of mindfulness training on counseling students' perceptions of stress. *Mindfulness*, 6(2), pp.159–169.

Freud, S. (1930) Civilization and its discontents. *SE XI* (57–146). London: Hogarth Press.

Garrote-Caparrós, E., Bellosta-Batalla, M., Moya-Albiol, L. and Cebolla, A. (2021). Effectiveness of mindfulness-based interventions on psychotherapy processes: A systematic review. *Clinical Psychology & Psychotherapy*, 29(3), pp.783–798.

Garrote-Caparrós, E., Lecuona, Ó., Bellosta-Batalla, M., Moya-Albiol, L. and Cebolla, A. (2022). Efficacy of a mindfulness and compassion-based intervention in psychotherapists and their patients: Empathy, symptomatology, and mechanisms of change in a randomized controlled trial. *Psychotherapy*, 59(4), pp.616–628.

Goldberg, S.B., Lam, S.U., Britton, W.B. and Davidson, R.J. (2022). Prevalence of meditation-related adverse effects in a population-based sample in the United States. *Psychotherapy Research*, 32 (3), pp.291–305.

Goyal, M., Singh, S., Sibinga, E.M.S., Gould, N.F., Rowland-Seymour, A., Sharma, R., Berger, Z., Sleicher, D., Maron, D.D., Shihab, H.M., Ranasinghe, P.D., Linn, S., Saha, S., Bass, E.B. and Haythornthwaite, J.A. (2014). Meditation programs for psychological stress and well-being. *JAMA Internal Medicine*, 174(3), p.357.

Grepmair, L., Mitterlehner, F., Loew, T. and Nickel, M. (2007a). Promotion of mindfulness in psychotherapists in training: Preliminary study. *European Psychiatry*, 22(8), pp.485–489.

Grepmair, L., Mitterlehner, F., Loew, T., Bachler, E., Rother, W. and Nickel, M. (2007b). Promoting mindfulness in psychotherapists in training influences the treatment results of their patients: A randomized, double-blind, controlled study. *Psychotherapy and Psychosomatics*, 76(6), pp.332–338.

Hemanth, P. and Fisher, P. (2014). Clinical psychology trainees' experiences of mindfulness: An interpretive phenomenological analysis. *Mindfulness*, 6(5), pp.1143–1152.

Hopkins, A. and Proeve, M. (2013). Teaching mindfulness-based cognitive therapy to trainee psychologists: Qualitative and quantitative effects. *Counselling Psychology Quarterly*, 26(2), pp.115–130.

Hunt, C.A., Goodman, R.D., Hilert, A.J., Hurley, W. and Hill, C.E. (2021). A mindfulness-based compassion workshop and pre-session preparation to enhance therapist effectiveness in psychotherapy: A pilot study. *Counselling Psychology Quarterly*, 35(3), pp.546–561.

Ivanovic, M., Swift, J.K., Callahan, J.L. and Dunn, R. (2015). A multisite pre/post study of mindfulness training for therapists: The impact on session presence and effectiveness. *Journal of Cognitive Psychotherapy*, 29(4), pp.331–342.

Kabat-Zinn, J. (2013) *Full Catastrophe Living: Using the Wisdom of Your Body and Mind to Face Stress, Pain, and Illness*. Revised and Updated Edition. New York: Bantam Books.

Kalmar, J., Bressler, C., Gruber, E., Baumann, I., Vonderlin, E., Bents, H., Heidenreich, T. and Mander, J. (2024). Mindfulness skills in trainee child and adolescent psychotherapists: Exploring the effects of mindfulness-based workshops in a mixed-methods study. *Counselling and Psychotherapy Research*, 24(1), pp.154–168.

Keane, A. (2013). The influence of therapist mindfulness practice on psychotherapeutic work: A mixed-methods study. *Mindfulness*, 5(6), pp.689–703.

Lalor, J. and Khoshfetrat, A. (2023). An examination of the association between mindfulness and compassion for others in psychotherapists: A mediating role of self-compassion. *Counselling and Psychotherapy Research*. https://onlinelibrary.wiley.com/doi/10.1002/capr.12735

Latorre, C., Leppma, M., Platt, L.F., Shook, N. and Daniels, J. (2021). The relationship between mindfulness and self-compassion for self-assessed competency and self-efficacy of psychologists-in-training. *Training and Education in Professional Psychology*, 17(2), pp.213–220.

Lutz, A., Jha, A.P., Dunne, J.D. and Saron, C.D. (2015). Investigating the phenomenological matrix of mindfulness-related practices from a neurocognitive perspective. *American Psychologist*, 70(7), pp.632–658.

Mahasi, S. (2016). *Manual of Insight*. Massachusetts: Wisdom Publications.

Matko, K. and Sedlmeier, P. (2019). What is meditation? Proposing an empirically derived classification system. *Frontiers in Psychology*, 10, p.2276.

Mccollum, E.E. (2014). *Mindfulness for Therapists : Practice for the Heart*. New York: Routledge, Taylor & Francis Group.

Michalak, J., Steinhaus, K. and Heidenreich, T. (2018). (How) do therapists use mindfulness in their clinical work? A study on the implementation of mindfulness interventions. *Mindfulness*, 11(2), pp.401–410.

Millon, G. and Halewood, A. (2015). Mindfulness meditation and countertransference in the therapeutic relationship: A small-scale exploration of therapists' experiences using grounded theory methods. *Counselling and Psychotherapy Research*, 15(3), pp.188–196.

Montero-Marin, J., Allwood, M., Ball, S., Crane, C., De Wilde, K., Hinze, V., Jones, B., Lord, L., Nuthall, E., Raja, A., Taylor, L., Tudor, K., Blakemore, S.-J., Byford, S., Dalgleish, T., Ford, T., Greenberg, M.T., Ukoumunne, O.C., Williams, J.M.G. and Kuyken, W. (2022). School-based mindfulness training in early adolescence: What works, for whom and how in the MYRIAD trial? *Evidence Based Mental Health*, 25(3), pp.117–124.

Moore, P. (2008). Introducing mindfulness to clinical psychologists in training: An experiential course of brief exercises. *Journal of Clinical Psychology in Medical Settings*, 15(4), pp.331–337.

Nash, J.D. and Newberg, A. (2013). Toward a unifying taxonomy and definition for meditation. *Frontiers in Psychology*, 4:2206, pp.464–499.

Nash, J.D. and Newberg, A.B. (2023). An updated classification of meditation methods using principles of taxonomy and systematics. *Frontiers in Psychology*, 13:1062535, pp.01–20.

Purser, R. (2019). *McMindfulness: How Mindfulness Became the New Capitalist Spirituality*. London: Repeater.

Reddy, J.S.K. and Roy, S. (2019). Understanding meditation based on the subjective experience and traditional goal: Implications for current meditation research. *Frontiers in Psychology*, 10:1827, pp.01–09.

Rimes, K.A. and Wingrove, J. (2010). Pilot study of mindfulness-based cognitive therapy for trainee clinical psychologists. *Behavioural and Cognitive Psychotherapy*, 39(2), pp.235–241.

Ryan, A., Safran, J.D., Doran, J.M. and Muran, J.C. (2012). Therapist mindfulness, alliance and treatment outcome. *Psychotherapy Research*, 22(3), pp.289–297.

Segal, Z.V., Williams, J.M.G. and Teasdale, J.D. (2013). *Mindfulness-Based Cognitive Therapy for Depression*, 2nd Edition. New York: The Guilford Press.

Shapiro, S.L., Brown, K.W. and Biegel, G.M. (2007). Teaching self-care to caregivers: Effects of mindfulness-based stress reduction on the mental health of therapists in training. *Training and Education in Professional Psychology*, 1(2), pp.105–115.

Shonin, E. and Van Gordon, W. (2014). Managers' experiences of meditation awareness training. *Mindfulness*, 6(4), pp.899–909.

Siegel, D.J. (2010). *The Mindful Therapist: A Clinician's Guide to Mindsight and Neural Integration*. New York: W.W. Norton & Co.

Sparby, T. and Sacchet, M.D. (2022). Defining meditation: Foundations for an activity-based phenomenological classification system. *Frontiers in Psychology*, 12:795077, pp.1–16.

Spinelli, C., Wisener, M. and Khoury, B. (2019). Mindfulness training for healthcare professionals and trainees: A meta-analysis of randomized controlled trials. *Journal of Psychosomatic Research*, 120, pp.29–38.

Swift, J.K., Callahan, J.L., Dunn, R., Brecht, K. and Ivanovic, M. (2017). A randomized-controlled crossover trial of mindfulness for student psychotherapists. *Training and Education in Professional Psychology*, 11(4), pp.235–242.

Taylor, G.B., Vasquez, T.S., Kastrinos, A., Fisher, C.L., Puig, A. and Bylund, C.L. (2022). The adverse effects of meditation-interventions and mind-body practices: A systematic review. *Mindfulness,* 13, pp.1839–1856.

Rodriguez Vega, B., Melero-Llorente, J., Bayon Perez, C., Cebolla, S., Mira, J., Valverde, C. and Fernández-Liria, A. (2013). Impact of mindfulness training on attentional control and anger regulation processes for psychotherapists in training. *Psychotherapy Research*, 24(2), pp.202–213.

Van Gordon, W., Shonin, E. and Griffiths, M.D. (2015). Towards a second generation of mindfulness-based interventions. *Australian & New Zealand Journal of Psychiatry*, 49(7), pp.591–592.

Walpola, P., Walpola, I. and Toneatto, T. (2022). A contemporary model for right mindfulness based on Theravada Buddhist texts. *Mindfulness*, 13, pp.2714–2728.

2 Taking a Deep Breath

The Breath and Breathing

The foundational meditation object in this book will be the breath which will be used to develop a general therapeutic mindset. I will be calling this mindset *the meditation frame* which is analogous to the psychotherapeutic frame established for the purpose of delivering therapy. Other meditation objects will be focussed on in later chapters in order to develop specific mindsets related to certain therapeutic modalities. I will explain aspects of the breath as they relate to meditation through four lenses:

- Physiological – The mechanisms involving the human body
- Psychological – Those phenomena arising from the mind relating to the mental and emotional content relating to meditation
- Neuroscientific – Concerning the brain, spinal cord and peripheral nervous system
- Using metaphorical language – Bringing a more symbolic way of relating to the more abstract phenomena that occur when meditating that do not fit into the first three lenses.

I give all these descriptions as different aspects of these explanations will resonate more with some readers than others. These four lenses will also be used throughout the book, with the different meditation techniques, which use objects other than the breath.

DOI: 10.4324/9781003382959-2

Physiological explanations are particularly powerful as they are phenomena which are observable within our own bodies. They provide a bottom-up approach to meditation where we think about how sensory stimuli might shape perceptions. Psychological descriptions fit well into the practice of psychotherapy, which is primarily a psychological discipline. Neuroscientific evidence points towards some of the underlying physical mechanisms occurring in the central and peripheral nervous systems, which are related to the psychological and physiological experience. This might appeal more to those readers who may be sceptical of meditation given its roots in religious and spiritual traditions and those who find the evidence base of neuroscience to be more appealing given it being more directly based on a physical aspect of the human body and therefore perceived as more empirical. There are, of course, issues with all three of these approaches in relation to the subjective experience of meditation. However, I feel they all build up to a helpful picture of why and how meditation operates. For this reason, I find the aforementioned metaphorical descriptions helpful in thinking about meditation and the breath with more symbolic language.

I initially found the more scientific understanding of meditation and the breath helpful to inform the range of experiences I had when focussing and using the breath to establish my meditation practice. Once I became more experienced, more metaphorical understandings, have helped to tackle some of the obstacles I have come up against and gave more colour to what otherwise can be quite a mechanistic description of what is experienced as less ordered and predictable. Thinking in a more symbolic way has helped to deepen my meditation practice as I have become less interested in the whys of experience and more focussed on what might be occurring, be that in terms of the physical sensations, emotional responses and thoughts and the effects of changes in the way I relate to them. I have taken a more phenomenological approach in this way. For example, with breath meditation, I had knowledge through my medical training of the physiological and neuroscientific processes that occur in the process of respiration. Therefore, I could sense a great deal of the physical processes that were occurring in my body, however, I struggled to make sense of the many meditation instructions around making use of the breath to bring about a calmer mindset or to bring more focus to the mind. It was by using symbolic descriptions of breath energy, which I was initially very resistant towards, that have helped me to break free from some of the more mechanistic scientific descriptors and develop a more meaningful relationship with my breath. This has allowed me to make a stronger connection between my mind, body, emotional world and capacity to form relationships in my therapeutic work and beyond.

The breath is utilised for a number of reasons. It is easily accessible and constantly present. The breath is probably the most integrated physiological phenomena in the body in the way that it is associated with a whole range of metabolic, psychological, affective, cognitive and physical processes (Del Negro, Funk and Feldman, 2018). That consequentially means that altering the breath has a wide range and depth of effects on different aspects of the mind and body. The breath sits on the cusp between the conscious and unconscious. The autonomic process of breathing continues regardless of intentional awareness but can also be consciously altered through the somatic or voluntary nervous system. The connection between emotional states and the body can be readily accessed through the breath. The nature of the breath will change depending on the emotional state; for example, the speed of the breath – hyperventilation when anxious and slower when calm. However, this works both ways and when the breath is intentionally changed it has an effect on emotional states. *Taking a deep breath* is a well-known expression describing how best to prepare for a stressful experience, or to regroup when feeling anxious. Using slow and measured breathing can reduce anxiety and is a well-known and effective grounding technique for when people feel panicked (Vlemincx, Van Diest and Van den Bergh, 2016). There is much more going on in the respiratory system and its consequential effects when controlling the breath that we will be able to explore and utilise during meditation (Zaccaro et al., 2018).

The Sigh and Slow Breathing

There are connections between the involvement of the nervous system, physiology of breathing and emotional experience. One way this is mediated is through respiratory sinus arrhythmia, a normal variation in heart rate occurring during the respiratory cycle, which is connected to the balance between the sympathetic and parasympathetic nervous systems. We can consciously intercept and alter this normal physiological process by adjusting our breathing to change the frequency of our heart rate and blood pressure levels, this having knock-on effects on our emotional state too. When we inhale, the heart rate and blood pressure increases and when breathing out it decreases. You can notice this yourself right now while reading this book. First, feel your pulse with the pads of two of your fingers either on your neck by your larynx or wrist at the base of your thumb. Get a sense of the pulse rate and then monitor it as you slowly breath in and out. You should notice a faster rate on the in breath and slower on the outbreath after trying it out for 5--10 cycles. The difference is more pronounced in younger and fitter people. The change in heart rate and blood pressure occurs due to the pressure changes in the chest between inspiration and expiration and the expansion and contraction of the chest through the breathing cycle. This then affects the blood flow to the heart and specialised pressure receptors in blood vessels, called baroreceptors. Baroceptors interact with the autonomic nervous system so that when breathing in, sympathetic activation leads to an increase in heart rate and blood pressure and vice versa when breathing out due to the parasympathetic nervous system. The function of respiratory sinus arrhythmia is thought to be either so that the amount of air going in and out of the lungs at each stage of respiration is matched by blood flow to optimise the exchange of oxygen and carbon dioxide (Ito et al., 2006) or it serves to minimise the amount of energy the heart uses to keep levels of carbon dioxide in the blood at healthy levels (Ben-Tal, Shamailov and Paton, 2012).

The autonomic nervous system includes two arms – the previously mentioned sympathetic, colloquially known as the flight or fight system, part of which causes the release of adrenaline (epinephrine is the same name derived from the Greek instead of Latin), and the parasympathetic, sometimes referred to as the rest or digest system, which is mostly mediated through the vagal nervous system. We can broadly think of activation of the parasympathetic system to be more favourable when working as a therapist, although many will have experienced moments of activation of the sympathetic system when fighting or flighting is not required due to heightened anxiety. We will see how manipulation of the breath can help to change and manage these systems.

By understanding this connection between the breath and the autonomic nervous system, we can see how, by reducing the length of the inspiratory phase compared to the expiratory phase, we can increase the parasympathetic response to slow down the heart rate and reduce blood pressure. The consequence of this is to bring about more calm and relaxation in quite an immediate way. Likewise, by extending the inspiratory phase, we can increase the heart rate and blood pressure. This can be helpful, for example, if feeling particularly drowsy, tired or the mind is feeling dull.

Breathing with an extended expiratory phase and repeating is known as cyclic sighing, a physiological sigh or, simply, as I will call it from here on in, a sigh. It has been shown to be an effective technique to improve mood, reduce anxiety and decrease breathing rate when compared to other breathwork techniques (Balban et al., 2023). This first part of the sigh involves taking a deep breath followed by a second shorter inhalation to fully inflate the lungs. The second in breath is advised as the lungs are not akin to two balloons but rather have approximately 480 million alveoli, which are tiny air sacs where the exchange of oxygen and carbon dioxide into the bloodstream occurs (Ochs et al., 2004). The second inhalation reinflates any of these many air sacs which might have collapsed during periods of more relaxed breathing, allowing for a greater amount of gas exchange to occur increasing the efficiency of the lungs. This is then followed by an elongated outbreath. I will often teach people a sigh as a powerful breathing technique to use in heightened states of anxiety or panic. Box breathing is another effective breathing technique in this way albeit a bit more lengthy. I detail how to practice box breathing in the *Other Complementary Techniques* chapter near the end of the book. Sighs have been shown to be psychological and physiological resetters associated with reduced anxiety and muscle tension (Vlemincx et al., 2016). For this reason, sighs will be used at the beginning of each meditation technique described in this book. Not only do they quickly help to bring about physical and psychological relaxation, but they demarcate a meditation as a different state of mind and body from just sitting down in a usual way – providing a ritualised start to a meditation session.

In addition to manipulating the breathing cycle, there is also some evidence that another way to increase the activity of the vagal parasympathetic arm of the autonomic system is by introducing a low-pitched humming sound on the exhalation phase. This is also known as a yogic breathing technique called Bhramari Pranayama in Sanskrit, meaning bumblebee breath in English. Probably one of the most cliched images of someone's meditation might have them sitting in a lotus position, hands on knee, palms up humming *om* with a low-pitched hum. However, it has been found that using a low frequency humming there has a similar effect to other meditation techniques when measured with an electroencephalogram (EEG) (Vialatte et al., 2009). There is a decrease in blood pressure and heart rate implying a parasympathetic response (Pramanik, Pudasaini and Prajapati, 2010), an increase in pulmonary function (Kuppusamy et al., 2017) and a general decrease in stress (Trivedi et al., 2023). Studies suggest that the humming significantly increases levels of nitrous oxide in the paranasal sinuses which can increase ventilation and gas exchange mediating the above effects (Lundberg, 2008; Weitzberg and Lundberg, 2002). This humming technique could be experimented with while exhaling in the initial stages of meditation or just generally as a grounding technique to see if it is something that can bring about additional relaxation.

Aside from the sigh, slow breathing techniques used in meditation have a variety of physiological benefits. Slow breathing is defined as a rate of 4–10 breaths per minute where the normal range is generally 10–20 for healthy adults. I find that when meditating my respiratory rate generally slows to this rate fairly quickly, especially after taking three sighs. By breathing slowly, there is more effective transport of air in and out of the lungs as the alveoli are more available to transport oxygen and carbon dioxide between the blood and lungs (Bernardi et al., 1998). Slow breathing techniques have been shown to have both cardiovascular and respiratory benefits with improvements to asthma (Burgess et al., 2011) and high blood pressure (Li et al., 2018).

While we have so far thought about the breath and the sensations being experienced from this more material and physiological perspective, sometimes a more metaphorical explanation may resonate more with others or offer more meaning to what might be experienced. This folds into those more spiritual traditions from where most meditation methods derive. Interestingly, the etymology of the word *spiritual* is the same as *respiratory* as it has to do with the breath, such is the recognition of how the breath has a unique relationship with the spirit or essence of a person. It is this connection with religious or metaphysical beliefs, which I think is due to the conscious/unconscious and autonomic/somatic axis associated with the breath. I acknowledge the concepts of qi from Chinese traditions of Tao and qi gong, prana in Hinduism or the practice of yoga, and to an extent, historical European concepts of the four humours are parallel to this idea, but writing this book from a secular and scientific perspective, I will eschew these religious traditions.

In the spirit of this idea using more symbolic language, the breath can be conceptualised in this different way. We can think of a movement of energy into and through the body as physically the movement of air, but also consequentially as the gas exchange occurring in the lungs and a refreshing energetic flow of movement as the oxygen is delivered to each cell in the body through the blood. By considering this breath energy, one can engender alternative physical and emotional responses. Therefore, you can alter the manner of breathing and by doing so effect a change in the spread of this breath energy from the sensations of inhalation and exhalation radiating from the chest to the peripheries. Taking the effects of the sigh in this way we could consider altering this spread of energy to something more calming and relaxing. While a materialistic explanation is one of changes to heart rate, blood pressure and the autonomic nervous system, something more metaphorical involving the conception of the breath energy pervading throughout the whole body might make more sense in terms of the experience of relaxing and the flow of these buzzing or tingling sensations. When considering changing the way we perceive the breath as more than the physical movement of gases and the consequential physiological and psychological changes, it can help to change the perception of uncomfortable sensations, pains and stressful psychological states that can arise in meditation. If we think of them as purely physical processes, it can be harder to imagine how they might change. Symbolic thinking opens up a different way of relating to the mind and body.

We will explore these techniques more in the troubleshooting section, but broadly speaking, they speak to how meditation can bring a greater understanding of the importance of understanding our influence in the perception of the environment and relationships deriving from our own attitudes rather than solely in the impact of the external on our inner world. The use of symbolism can be analogous to how metaphor is used in psychotherapy by clients and therapists alike as a means of conceptualising affect through language and to understand without the potentially overwhelming direct experience. I appreciate that without having practised meditation much, these ideas may seem a bit fanciful to some, so feel free to put them to one side if they do not resonate. However, after becoming more familiar with the breath and consequentially other objects in the context of meditation, it might be helpful to return to these ideas.

Beyond the Breath

Thinking beyond the breath, we can notice these changes in heart rate and blood pressure in our bodies resulting from this difference in breathing when we focus our attention on bodily sensations. It is possible to not just notice the heart rate in our chest or when putting our fingers on the carotid artery on our necks but also when sitting still. You can also feel the flow of blood at multiple spots, such as the head bobbing slightly, or in the arms, hands, legs and feet. When limbs are bent such as if sitting cross-legged or when resting the hand on the knee a pulse can be felt. Likewise, blood pressure changes can be detected due to the cycle of breathing, on the level of physical relaxation in sensations at the peripheries when pressure decreases or a more intense sensations when blood pressure increases. This is more apparent *in extremis,* such as moments of high stress when the results of the sympathetic nervous system and adrenaline result in this fight or flight experience. By bringing attention to the body and training ourselves to notice more, we can become increasingly sensitive to the feeling of blood flow, the heartbeat and the movement of air during respiration, which are three of the main bodily movements occurring when sitting still. In addition, the body will subtly adjust itself to maintain an upright position when seated or standing due to the systems of balance and proprioception – the sense allowing us to be aware of the position and movement of different parts of the body. These sensations form the content of experience for body-based meditations such as the body scan, where the object is not just the breath but different sensations within the body.

The subtle body can be used as a way to describe the less apparent experience of bodily sensations that can arise when attention is more focussed on specific areas of the body as opposed to the more gross sensations of pressure, pain or large movements that are more apparent in our everyday levels of experiencing the sensory inputs of touch or proprioception. These sensations are often, though not always restricted, to a sort of tingling, buzzing or bubbling sensation. We can observe this by bringing our attention to say our thumb on the left hand and notice any feeling that might be occurring there. There might be pulsing from the blood flowing, a slight sensation of touch where the thumb is against another object, or maybe you can detect these other more subtle sensations mentioned above. Practices such as body scanning, which we will explore later in the book, sweep the attention through the surface of the body and any sensations within, noticing these sensations and any others that might be occurring. These sensations are constantly happening, we just do not notice them when our attention is not focussed there. While there have been some attempts to marry the idea of this subtle body with neuroscience, it has as yet to gain much credibility (Loizzo, 2016). We will cover in more detail a body scanning meditation in the *Body-Centred Psychotherapy – Somatic Perspectives* chapter.

The breath will be one of the meditation objects used. With every technique, I have suggested that you begin by taking three sighs before exploring how a specific way of focussing on the breath. The breath can then be used to establish a specific mindset which can incorporate the whole practice, or in other chapters, we will use that mindset to transfer awareness to other meditation objects. For the psychodynamic approach these secondary objects will include the experiences of countertransference and reveries. In person-centred counselling we will develop the experience of unconditional positive regard (UPR) using a process of focussing on certain visualisations and generating an effective experience. We will use the imagination to conjure up a situation where it is easier to generate the feeling of UPR before extending it to other situations. Other meditations will use repetition of a phrase or question as a self-enquiry similar to a mantra, and there will be other visualisation exercises to bring about the specific mindsets for mentalisation-based therapy. There will also be descriptions of a range of other complementary techniques including box breathing, walking meditation, a combination between breath meditation and body scanning, progressive muscle relaxation and specific meditations using listening and looking. We will also explore how some of these meditation practices can be integrated into everyday activities, specifically when working as a therapist be that with a client in the consultation room, before seeing clients or afterwards.

A General Therapeutic Stance

While the meditation method to *Establish The Meditation Frame* is the starting point for all the techniques that I have suggested, it can be used independently to foster the characteristics that are common to all therapists. These common factors, as described below, are especially important to psychotherapists who work integratively with a range of models, drawing on the strengths and relevance of each approach depending on the client who presents to them. Some research shows that regardless of technique, it is the quality of the therapeutic relationship which moderates the outcome of the treatment, that different psychotherapies have generally similar effectiveness, and that it is the characteristics of the client and therapist which affects results (Castonguay and Beutler, 2006; Livesley, 2007; Norcross, 2011). This is not to talk down therapists who use a single approach indeed I work as a psychodynamic psychotherapist, but rather draw us to the importance of developing this capacity for a strong therapeutic relationship, underpinned by these common factors.

Meditation can be used to enhance the capacity of the psychotherapist to develop these factors many of which can be inferred from the many neurological changes seen with a meditation practice. Generally speaking, meditation changes are observed through the changes in self-awareness, emotional regulation and attention control with corresponding structural changes in the brain, including the anterior cingulate cortex, prefrontal cortex, posterior cingulate cortex, insula, amygdala and striatum. This long list points towards the myriad effects that meditation has (Tang, Hölzel and Posner, 2015). The key to self-awareness and relating information to oneself incorporates the faculties of mind-wandering and self-referential processing. These processes are connected to default mode network activation which is related to ruminating, a significant feature of depression. It has been found that areas of the default mode network are less active in experienced meditators. It is thought this is the corresponding neurological correlate for the effects of meditation in reducing depressive symptoms as there is a reduction in rumination through the regulation of this mind-wandering and self-referential processing. We can see how this mechanism can also enhance a therapeutic mindset and the relationship with the general therapeutic stance below to bring about more focus. It has been found that a month's meditation practice can trigger an increase in connectivity between the default mode network with the salience network and central executive network, a triple network which is proposed as a way to explain how the many changes seen in the many smaller areas of the brain might operate together in large scale networks (Bremer et al., 2022). The inner workings of the brain and its relationship to the very diverse effects of meditation are yet to be fully explored, instead being broadly mapped onto these more general outcomes. Similarly, books written on the topic of psychotherapy and meditation have focussed on more broad common factors (Alper, 2016; McCollum, 2014; Siegel, 2010). We can explore how meditation can foster these common factors, as well as the more psychoanalytic perspectives of holding and containing, for a general therapeutic stance:

Focussed Attention and Listening

By listening to ourselves in meditation under the light of alertness and noticing all that is occurring in our minds which might usually pass us by, our capacity to listen to others also increases. In addition, the development of a focus and concentration which allows for less distraction and undesired mind wandering lets us observe and notice what might be occurring for ourselves and clients. Simply the act of being truly present and alongside a client can have a great therapeutic effect, especially for clients who may not have had anyone in their lives to think with and take seriously their inner world.

This has also been shown in various studies – alerting, orientating and conflict monitoring attention systems were assessed on groups either doing an MBSR or concentrative meditation course. Interestingly, the two groups enhanced different types of attention pointing towards the connection between meditation technique and mindset (Jha, Krompinger and Baime, 2007). It has also been shown how sustained attention with increased perceptual sensitivity and vigilance can be developed if a more intensive meditation practice is practised (MacLean et al., 2010).

Patience and Robustness

The process of mindfulness – remembering to bring the attention back to the object of meditation – being employed repeatedly, even though at times being immensely frustrating or in the face of mental and physical discomfort, delivers an increase in our capacity for patience and the development of robustness. It can be a great relief for a client to be with someone who is able to be patient and thoughtful with them rather than responding in ways that people in previous relationships have or indeed have with themselves. Likewise, the capacity to relate to environmental stressors to be compassionate and patient with ourselves brings a greater resilience against both compassion fatigue and burnout, which, as in every caring profession, is an ever present risk. This is due to the nature of exposure to mental distress in the work itself, the desire to be able to support others with this and the types of people who tend to find themselves in these vocations who may be more likely to put others before their own needs.

Self-Awareness

Simply by noticing just how much the mind is out of what we might feel to be our control as well as getting in touch with parts of the mind and body that had previously been obscured can facilitate an increase in self-awareness. So, for example, one study showed that the more experience a meditator has, the higher their introspective accuracy in tactile sensitivity while practising a body scanning meditation (Fox et al., 2012). We can deduce that this can extend to other realms of experience depending on the meditation object, such as cognitive or emotional. This self-awareness can be brought to the consultation room by using our countertransference as insight into a client's state of mind and prevent acting in on these experiences. Meditation also offers, through an increase in self-awareness, the potential for self-development which can be undertaken on our own terms without potentially onerous financial or time commitments from ourselves or others. This can be particularly refreshing in the psychotherapy profession, where expectations of continuous professional development can sometimes feel like more of a burden than an aid or when more supervision or personal therapy is given as the answer to a clinical question.

Reacting with Thought Rather than Action

By keeping with the meditation object, despite difficulties that might arise and being creative in the process to overcome discomfort and the myriad other challenges that arise can confer a greater tolerance for thought rather than action. Through repetitive mindfulness, we can train ourselves to be empathic instead of intolerant, creating space for thoughtfulness. This can correspond to working with clients and not reaching for false reassurance or advice, when listening and reflection might be a more clinically effective, albeit potentially uncomfortable response. Likewise, clients who might be more challenging to be with the action of referring out or ending a therapy perceived to be not making progress by a therapist may be supplanted by a more reflective, empathic and thoughtful presence.

Empathy and Compassion

Getting more in touch with the inner world and the challenges therein can give insight and therefore empathy towards the struggles a client might bring. Using specific techniques to develop an emotional capacity of empathy can also enhance the innate potential of all to bring into the consultation room. Mindfully returning to the meditation object with an empathic attitude towards ourselves, rather than frustration, can further increase this faculty. Many clients may never have experienced a calm, thoughtful and empathic presence. Meditation can aid greatly in making that potential in the therapist as strong as possible.

An eight-week meditation course was found to increase a compassionate response to suffering by more than five times (Condon et al., 2013). Using a specific loving-kindness and compassion focussed meditation backed up these findings (Hofmann, Grossman and Hinton, 2011). This specific meditation method, which has been adapted for the chapter on *Person-Centred Counselling – Unconditional Positive Regard* even found positive effects on the immune and endocrine systems (Pace et al., 2009) as well as enhancing brain areas involved in emotional processing and empathy, such as the insula and the anterior cingulate cortex (Lutz et al., 2008, 2009).

Boundaries

The establishment of boundaries in therapy is highly important and falls within the realm of those ethical values to which all therapists will subscribe. Boundaries create an atmosphere of predictability and safety serving to define the relationship with the client and creating a framework for treatment. They have multiple functions to set the expectations of therapy, including establishing trust, the limits of confidentiality and self-disclosure. Boundary crossings depart from commonly accepted practices that could potentially benefit the client and more severe boundary violations occur when a therapist misuses their power resulting in harm or exploitation to a client, forming a serious breach that could be unethical or illegal. These crossings and violations occur more commonly than probably thought by the general population and definitely more commonly than should be expected. They can be compounded when dual relationships occur – where the therapist has a relationship with a client outside of the and with the added challenge of the consultation room, often compounded by working in small communities.

There are many reasons for therapists to cross boundaries, including putting short-term needs and desires of the therapist or client ahead of the long-term interests of the client, such as with inappropriate gifts, gossiping or overly intimate relationships. Given how emotionally involved it can be working with clients, for some therapists, the desire to help can be so strong that it can be challenging to maintain appropriate boundaries. The ways in which some clients relate to others make it very challenging to maintain boundaries, especially in forensic settings. Therefore, it is crucial for therapists to keep boundaries in mind and when something unexpected or emotionally powerful is experienced, there be enough space in our minds to be able to pause and think with clients about what has occurred instead of taking action, be that in a knowing way or unconsciously.

Meditation can help develop a robust mindset whereby the practice of staying alert and noticing what is happening in the room with a client, maintaining mindfulness to bring the mind back when something unexpected happens and keeping ardency to stay true to boundaries and resist acting on any potential boundary crossings helps to maintain boundaries. This means that even if something unexpected occurs and perhaps a boundary has been crossed, we can still come back to it and think about it together with a client, thus potentially breaking a cycle of relating which a client can be so used to. Inevitably, there will be partial enactments especially when taking into consideration powerful countertransferential experiences. This will be discussed further in the chapter on *The Psychoanalytic Stance – Internal Listening*.

Holding

Donald Winnicott (1896–1971) was a British paediatrician and psychoanalyst who developed a number of psychoanalytic theories and practices which continue to be highly influential to this day. He was also well known due to his books written for lay audiences and radio programs that were broadcast in the United Kingdom. Winnicott developed the concept of the holding environment to show how a mother contributed to the development of their baby through an ordinary loving relationship. He then extended this concept into the consulting room extrapolating how the therapist relates and supports clients.

Holding is predicated by what Winnicott called the mother's primary maternal preoccupation whereby the mother is in a sense at one with the baby so as not to overwhelm them with the presence of another and provide that environment which is necessary to support the psychic development of the baby. This is balanced by Winincott's concept of *the good enough mother*, that they need not be some kind of perfect parent, in fact, the child needs to experience their parents as imperfect as an important part of their growth. Such a concept can be readily updated to reflect more current parental expectations, with the potential to replace the mother with that of a father or other primary care giver.

Holding sums up that unique state of mind which a parent has in those early days with an infant which you might be familiar with yourself, or having observed with someone close to you. The holding environment provided by the parent then aids the development of the child before they can become more separate, managing their own difficulties and challenges a bit more independently. It aids the movement from "absolute dependence," through "relative dependence," "towards independence" (Winnicott, 1960).

Therefore, with a client, the therapist can embody this similar *good enough therapist* and offer a holding environment for the clients to be able to experience their distress in a safe empathic environment facilitated by all the above faculties. The holding allows the client to experience someone who is empathic and sensitive to their needs but also not suffocating, someone who can aid their development through first a dependence then individuation. This is also achieved with a safe and consistent environment with someone who is attuned to the client with a genuine and authentic connection to facilitate an emotional closeness. The holding environment is, therefore, a co-created intersubjective space which supports this process occurring over a period of time. While only in some somatic therapies would the therapist physically touch the client, the emotional and psychological environment being provided can be seen to be analogous to that of the parent with the infant, especially if this was something lacking for the client in their early life. It helps the client to process past experiences, build resilience, and develop healthier ways of relating to themselves and others.

Through meditation, we can see how these capacities can be developed and lead up to a person who might be able to provide this sort of environment. The meditation exercise *Establishing The Meditation Frame* below is in essence developing the capacities to provide this holding environment.

Containing

I find the concept of the therapist as a container in a relationship with a client (the contained) to be a most helpful way to conceptualise a fundamental mindset of the therapist across therapeutic modalities. Regardless of the way a therapist works I think it offers a basic position which encompasses a range of features that enable the therapeutic process.

Wilfred Bion (1897–1979) was a first world war veteran, doctor and psychoanalyst working mostly in London and California later in life. He was a pioneer in group dynamics and therapy especially in the treatment of people with psychosis. Bion also developed an epistemological theory of thinking. According to Bion, every individual has a need for a container who can take in and make sense of their emotional experiences. Like Winnicott (and indeed most of the early psychoanalysts like Sigmund Freud and Melanie Klein), Bion went back to the mother or primary care giver in their role with the infant to show this function at play. He denoted reverie as the mental function of the container as the mother with an infant and when drawing an equivalence to the role of the therapist with a client. The container refers to the therapist or any other significant figure in a person's life capable of providing a safe and supportive environment for emotional expression.

In the container-contained dynamic (Bion, 1962), the individual's emotional experiences and thoughts are referred to as the contained. It encompasses their unconscious anxieties, fears, desires, and other psychological contents. The container, on the other hand, represents the therapeutic or supportive presence that can take in and process these emotional experiences before delivering them back to the contained in a palatable form. Bion emphasised that the container's role is not simply to absorb or eliminate the contained material but rather to help the individual make meaning out of it. The container engages in a process of understanding and transforming the emotional experiences by providing containment, validation, empathy, and interpretation.

Often, one hears in therapeutic circles about something being contained by a therapist or caregiver in a way where it is implied the person's distress has been kept from being overwhelming, keeping it boundaried and prevented from spilling over. However, it is more than just managing the other's emotions and ensuring they are not overpowered by them. There is a process of taking in what the other is experiencing, processing it and then having digested it into a palatable form, communicating it back. Between parent and infant, this happens in a way whereby the communicating back can be through physical gestures, comforting song or another unconscious relating. If you have ever been with a baby who is upset, picked them up and soothed them, you will be familiar with that initial experience of feeling a bit panicked by their distress, perhaps with a fantasy that they will never calm down or if it has been going on for a long time some kind of angry experiences arising, disorganised thoughts and feelings. That is not to say you would act on this anger, but they tell us something about the level of distress which the baby needs to put into the parent in order to protect themselves from fully experiencing it. Through the process of meditation and developing those other features described above, we are able to develop this capacity to be a container who can take on, process and deliver back those raw and unprocessed emotional experiences that are yet to be transformed into meaningful thoughts.

It can be hard to get in touch with the experience of containing, yet through a meditation practice which is then brought into the consultation room, I have found this to be more immediate and noticeable both in the mental, emotional and physical experience. I have found the role of a container through reverie to be a most helpful concept and practice in processing and making sense of a client's distress and oftentimes potentially bewildering presentation.

Through becoming more familiar with our own internal processes in meditation outside of the consultation room as well as using techniques during and after sessions, which will be explored later in the book, I have found the common factors to become more familiar and accessible. The process of *Establishing The Meditation Frame* will serve to develop these general factors, before we go on to describe meditation techniques that are matched to more specific mindsets.

Establishing the Meditation Frame

Posture

The first step to regular meditation practice is to find a place where you might be able to practise regularly. This will make that area familiar each time you go to meditate and over time will help to create a habit associated with that location. That is not to say you cannot meditate elsewhere, but by not using, say your bed or chair at the kitchen table, which is usually reserved for other activities, the location will become strongly associated with meditation and, therefore, a habit. Ideally this would be indoors, in a location which does not have direct sunlight onto your face but also is not particularly dark so as to bring about drowsiness. You can meditate outdoors, but for a beginner there might be too many distractions.

I prefer the posture of sitting on the floor, as it is not a usual position for me to take so makes the very posture is immediately associated with the practice. There are a variety of different ways to sit. I find a position known as *Burmese style* sitting on a cushion to raise my hips up easiest. Here, both knees are placed on the floor with feet one in front of the other in the midline but not crossed over each other. For many years, I also sat half lotus with one foot on the thigh of the other, both knees were on the ground, sitting a cushion, or just kneeling on a meditation bench. These benches are widely available and can be good if you are not so flexible. Other styles include full lotus, where both feet are on the opposite hip requiring quite a lot of flexibility or cross legged sometimes with a cushion to rest knees on or simply kneeling while sitting on a cushion.

Sitting on the floor is not always possible or comfortable enough for everyone. So, sitting on a chair, as I did at a recent meditation retreat due to leg pain, lying down or even standing is also fine. My main issue with lying down is I associate it with sleeping and, therefore, will struggle not to drop off to sleep once I settle into meditation. If I stand, my feet tend to get tired of staying in one position without moving. Walking meditation is different in that it can be a meditation practice itself and I will outline that later in the book. For the purposes of the guided meditations, I will assume a sitting posture, but the instructions can be broadly adapted for lying, standing or sitting on a chair too. It is helpful to keep the same position for each meditation simply so that you then do not need to think a lot about your position and can focus on the meditation itself. Establish a position you can take relatively comfortably early on and then ask questions, such as *should my hands be in this way or that? Or how straight should my back be?* are not too much of a concern. It's important to note that there will never be a perfect position which will be completely comfortable and devoid of any itch or pressure point. Physical discomfort will inevitably arise, much of which is actually an expression of psychological stress but can be a real obstacle to practice. A lot of this can be dealt with within the meditation itself and we will discuss issues like this throughout the book as well as more fully in the *Troubleshooting* chapter. The guided meditation below will give more descriptions of the variations and guidance for posture beyond the sitting position.

Timing

A regular timeslot is also beneficial for the same reason as location. I prefer to meditate in the mornings as I am more of a lark and feel more awake and motivated earlier in the day. If you are an owl then you may be more alert in the evenings. I tend to find it more challenging after eating during the postprandial lull. As with so many factors in meditation, it is up to you to find what works. Regularity is more important than the length of time for one session of meditation. So, five minutes a day is more effective than one hour once a week. I find the effect is more cumulative in this way. If you are totally new to meditation, then starting with a five-minute meditation (or maybe even two if that proves too demanding) may be most appropriate and increasing it as is comfortable from there. Try to be realistic about what might be achievable, meditation can be hard work, but it is meant to be a reasonably relaxing and pleasurable experience overall. If you are finding it significantly uncomfortable then do flick forwards to the *Troubleshooting* section and see if you can address some of the challenges there. Equally, it may be a matter of having been a little too ambitious from the beginning and to dial back on the amount of time that it feels comfortable to sit. If you have ever undertaken a new physical exercise or learned to play an instrument, it can be much the same in how it can be exciting to read about and practice at the beginning, but taking on too much in the actual practice, too early on, may extinguish some of that enthusiasm quickly and create a reluctance associated with the practice. Therefore, start slowly and steadily increase from there.

We first set the intention of the meditation to remain for whichever length of time we choose. This intention is a function of ardency. You can easily find meditation timer apps to install on your phone which have unalarming chimes to indicate when the time is up. Alternatively, you can just use a regular alarm. This is to remove the temptation to clock watch. It is important to do your best to stay meditating for the intended timeslot even if things do become challenging. By staying the full length of time it gives a sense of satisfaction and achievement. If you get into the routine of stopping early, then it will reduce the resilience and effectiveness of the practice as a training.

The Mouth, Nose and Eyes

In all the breathing meditations, I would suggest breathing through your nose. First, it is generally more comfortable than mouth breathing, which can become very dry if continued for an extended period. There is also evidence that nasal breathing has a different effect on the central nervous system than mouth breathing in the amygdala and hippocampus, which is related to stress and anxiety management (Zelano et al., 2016) as well as a connection with increased alertness and learning (Perl et al., 2019). There is plenty of evidence that it is generally better to breathe through the nose than the mouth in any situation due to filtering out or foreign substances, humidifying air, increasing oxygen uptake and improving circulation. Prolonged mouth breathing also changes facial anatomy, altering the shape of the jaw with misaligned teeth. All of this is written about at length elsewhere (Nestor, 2022). If your nose is blocked for whatever reason, then do breathe through your mouth instead or both together. Of course, mouth breathing will happen soon enough anyway if the nose is blocked.

Some meditation traditions make a distinction between abdominal or diaphragmatic breathing, whereby only the diaphragm is doing the mechanical work of breathing, and chest or thoracic breathing, where the muscles of the chest wall and other accessory muscles are the driving forces in the movement of air into the lungs. I do find when more relaxed I am mostly breathing only using the diaphragm and some suggest that intentionally breathing in this way makes one more relaxed. Diaphragmatic breathing increases the efficiency of blood moving back to the heart due to the connection of the diaphragm with the vena cava, one of the main veins which brings blood to the heart (Byeon et al., 2012). Diaphragmatic breathing can also facilitate a slower respiratory rate, the benefits of which I have mentioned (Stromberg, Russell and Carlson, 2015), as well as providing a smoother breathing experience (Vostatek et al., 2013), which I generally find to be more conducive to reaching a more focussed mindset. That said, as with all of these variations, do experiment and find out what works best for you.

I prefer to meditate with my eyes shut as this removes distractions coming in and external stimulations as we turn our attention inwards. However, in some traditions, meditation is done with eyes open or partially open, and on occasion it can be helpful to partially open eyes if feeling drowsy or the mind is particularly agitated. In the *Other Complementary Techniques* chapter, I describe some meditations I call *looking* using coloured discs or a candle as an accessory or with a technique called *focussed noticing*, which all require eyes open.

Place

It can sometimes be hard to find a quiet place to meditate. In the past, I have used earplugs to block sound out. You could also use noise cancelling earphones, although I find they sometimes come with their own more subtle sounds due to movement as well as discomfort when worn for prolonged periods. Generally, complete silence is impossible and, if anything, if you can meditate with some background noise, it will help to develop your faculties of concentration and robustness anyway, although it can be challenging depending on the volume and nature of the noises. Be sure that you also will not be disturbed by anyone else in the vicinity calling for you and expecting a reply by letting them know you will be meditating quietly for however long you have set your timer.

Beginning

After taking the posture and setting our intentions, we will consciously try to put aside any of the main thoughts that might be present. Usually, this would be those things that we currently want to happen (or do not want to happen) and those things that are a source of stress in the external world. While they may very well work their way back into our minds, it is a useful step to take as it again helps to set the frame for meditation as we turn inwards and away from external desires or troubles. So, for example, we might be thinking about want we want to eat for dinner or be worried about how work or a relationship is going. By noticing these things are in the mind and consciously putting them to one side at the start of the meditation it can help to keep them at bay before focussing on the intention to meditate. After this, we will take a quick survey of our body and mind to bring about an awareness of what sort of situation we are in at the beginning of the meditation.

The meditation exercise below will establish the frame for all the meditations in this book. Take some time to become familiar with how you might feel most comfortable to practise and really establish what I call a home in the breath – somewhere familiar, comfortable, a source of increased self-sufficiency where you can adapt to different challenges that might arise. This home can become a refuge and a place to return to when the mind might become unsettled in the face of stress, others' distress or distraction. Familiarity with your breath and its relationship with your body and mind will be a core skill to develop for further meditation exercises. It is important to develop not just mindfulness to remember to stay with the breath but also alertness to really notice what is going on. This helps to develop the ability to change and develop the faculties of concentration and discernment, as well as drop those habits which might be interfering with practice as per your ardency. This is where this initial meditation might differ from a more non-judgemental, present moment and open awareness practice. We are trying to do something, to get the mind somewhere and using the breath to do that as well as focussing in on a particular part of the breath. If you can figure out what kind of breathing can support that mindset, then you will have gone some of the way to changing the way you relate to your mind and body, how you can become less reactive and more able to work with your experiences in a constructive manner. When focussing the mind with the breath, it is commonly advised to pick a specific location to focus the attention. Some meditation traditions, for example, take the tip of the nose and ends of the nostrils (Goenka, 1987), others the abdomen moving outwards and inwards (Mahasi, 2016) with each breath. I like to focus on my chest area, but it comes down to person preference. So, see if you can find a location that suits you, where you can establish that *home* in your breath, where it feels comfortable and you can return to when needing some nourishment and ease during meditation. That is why it can be so helpful to work on a firm foundation in meditation before practising other techniques proposed in the book, as you can always return to a place that is familiar to you, like a port in a storm.

Ending

As with every meditation session, it is helpful to spend a couple of minutes after emerging from the experience to review how things went. This act can help to consolidate the experience and give a rough measurement of change or progress. Some people find it helpful to document this either by keeping a log with dates and lengths of sittings or a journal to describe the experience qualitatively. There is a template for a meditation log and journal at the end of the book. Most meditation apps will provide the former. I prefer to do this within my own thoughts as I do not respond well to tracking, but I am conscious for many seeing a visual representation through the data of a log combined with the self-reflective function of a journal can be highly motivational. Initially, I think about the experience in terms of some general questions:

- ◆ Did I manage to remember to remain with the meditation object?
- ◆ Did I generate the aimed for mindset?
- ◆ What did the session feel like?
- ◆ How am I left feeling at the end of the session?

These are but a few questions we can ask ourselves. I prefer for things not to be too formulaic, but sometimes making things more formal can provide more structure for a reflection and for this reason, I have suggested additional questions for reflection at the end of each meditation exercise. Equally, you can simply write about whatever emerges in your thoughts and feelings.

Guided Meditation Exercise – Establishing the Frame and Exploring the Breath

Take your seated position, lying or standing, if you are unable. Try to keep things fairly symmetrical so your shoulders are in line with hips, nose in the midline. If on a chair, keep your legs square on with your feet firmly on the ground. Some people like to put a cushion beneath their feet or knees for comfort depending on their flexibility. Try to keep the back erect, but not so that you are holding an uncomfortable position. It is a balance between not being slumped so you start to become drowsy and not too tense in an upright position that will leave you feeling agitated.

Make sure your mouth is closed so you are breathing through your nose, assuming it is not blocked. Keep your tongue on the roof of your mouth, but not touching your front teeth which will aid in keeping the nasal airway more open. You can notice this difference by breathing through your nose with your tongue on the bottom of the mouth and the consequential sense of a narrowed nasal airway.

Try keeping your hands in a symmetrical way either on your knees face up or downwards, or palms facing upwards on top of each other. I find interlacing my fingers can feel somewhat tense. In whatever posture you have taken, now look out a few metres in front of you before slowly closing your eyes and turning your attention inwards.

Try to intentionally put aside some of the more immediate concerns that may be on your mind, things that you might be wanting or not, or things you may be worried about both related to your daily life and the meditation itself. Then set the intention to stay in this position for the time you have allotted for this meditation, this can be done using your inner voice saying something like *I will remain here for the full duration of the meditation*, or by imagining yourself finishing the session having kept to your intention.

Take a minute or two to do a quick survey of your mind and body. Notice what might be the main theme of thinking occurring in your mind at the moment. Perhaps there are thoughts about what might have been happening just now or concerns for the near or far future. Consider also your emotional state. What is your current overall mood and which affect might be predominate?

After surveying the mind, we will do the same with the body. Move your attention from the top of your head, to your neck, through each arm and hands, down your torso and then along each leg to your feet. Where you may notice tension try to relax, if you find yourself leaning towards one side or another, try to reach a place of balance in between. If you can feel some tension it might help to flex or slightly move the associated muscle and then relax it again. Notice the sensation of the pressure of your body where it meets itself, on your seated area and where your body makes contact with the ground, including feet or knees, depending on how you are seated.

We will then turn out attention towards the breath beginning with three sighs. Take a deep breath in through the nose relatively swiftly, once fully inhaled breath in a little bit more to fully inflate the chest, before very slowly exhaling until you have emptied your lungs of your breath. You can try a low frequency hum while exhaling and see if that makes the sigh more effective in bringing about calm and grounding yourself in the experience of the breath and body. Some people also prefer to breath out through their mouth when sighing. By pursing the lips together, this can slow down the exhalation phase. As we will be breathing through the nose for all the meditation methods, using the mouth makes the sigh more of a unique aspect of the practice, creating a ritual to signify the beginning of this phase of the meditation. Repeat this twice more to make a total of three sighs, paying attention to the difference in length between the quicker inhalation and slow exhalation. Perhaps you also feel some other sensations in your body some more apparent, others more subtle – the movement of the body and air with the breathing, a warmness or tingling in the limbs, a slowing of your heart rate and pulse in the peripheries, or a relaxation of tensions in the body.

Begin to allow the breath to settle in whichever way is comfortable at the moment. Start by noticing different features of the breath both between inhalation and exhalation and between different cycles of the breath. Are they:

♦ Long or short?
♦ Deep or shallow?
♦ Quick or slow?
♦ Smooth or rough?
♦ Consistent or inconsistent?
♦ Through the right nostril, the left or both?
♦ Warm or cool?

While noticing these different features of the breath, track the breath all the way from the most exterior part of the nostrils towards the back of the nose as it comes to our throat and down into our lungs. Notice not just the movement and sensations of the air but also that of the body. How when breathing in deeply, the chest and shoulders lift upwards and outwards and the abdomen expands. The reverse then occurs in exhalation – the abdomen moves inwards and the chest and shoulders move in and down. When breathing less deeply, perhaps there is enough air movement without engaging the chest and simply the diaphragm at the abdomen is moving. On exhalation we can follow the sensations of the breath from the base of the lungs and the reverse of before. We will now move to focus on one particular area, such as the tip of the nose, the abdomen moving in and out, around the centre of the chest, the throat trying to stay at this location for the rest of the session helping to establish a focussed concentration.

Every time the mind wanders off, we will bring our attention back to this more focussed part of the breath trying each time to catch our mind before it goes off into a full daydream. It is important to do this, being mindful, remembering to keep the breath in mind in a way which is gentle, a bit like redirecting a child who has wandered off course when walking down the road. Our habit is for the mind to wander and usually to follow it off like being caught in the flow of a river. If we respond in a harsh or annoyed way it will be hard to practise long term due to negative associations of frustration. For this reason, sometimes it can help to smile slightly or say to ourselves something simple along the lines of *oh the mind has wandered off again, let's bring ourselves back to the breath* with a little smile of recognition. By not associating strongly with the process, it does not become a solid part of our identities and then can be easier to manage. If we respond to ourselves in this gentle way, it also supports the development of empathy towards ourselves and others.

This process then continues. We follow the breath, alert to all the phenomena that are occurring, the mind wanders and mindfully we bring our attention back before focussing in again ardently aiming to maintain this focus.

To help keep the attention on the breath, we can try to make it a more pleasant and stimulating experience. See if you can change the way you breathe so that something like a warmth, a tingling sensation or just a general sense of comfort arises with the breath in the part of the breath we are focussed on. I find breathing more shallowly, slowly and smoothly can bring about a more calming experience. However, experiment with the breath and see if you too can find a place in your breath which is more pleasant. We are creating a home in the breath where we can always come back to, somewhere comfortable which can hold our attention.

As time goes on, see if you can maintain your focus on this area and when your mind does wander, if you can bring it back at a shorter interval. If you find your mind is particularly lethargic then try breathing a bit rougher to give yourself something more solid to be aware of or extend the length of the inhalation and have a shorter exhalation – the opposite of the sigh. You can also go back to taking some sighs as at the beginning if you find your mind to be very restless and bouncing back and forth between different ideas. Try to breathe slower and longer to calm things down or to breathe out slower to extend the phase of exhalation and breathe in faster. However, different ways of breathing might have their own effects for you and see if you can experiment and develop what works best for you. If you can develop more awareness of this connection between the breath, the body and the field of emotional experience, it will serve to further build up the breath as a more solid and reliable home, as well as give you a whole new field of experience to explore and bring into your everyday and professional life.

Continue with the meditation, focussing on the specific place you have chosen, be that the tip of your nose, your chest or abdomen, for the full length of the timer and when you feel ready, gradually open your eyes, relax and stretch your body and bring back your awareness to your environment.

Some questions on which to reflect:

◆ Were you surprised by just how much of the content of the mind is filtered out in our everyday experiences, which you are exposed to when sitting quietly?
◆ What was it like to remain alert on one specific area of the breath and use mindfulness to bring the attention back when it drifted?
◆ Did you notice the effect of the breath on any aspects of your experience?
◆ Could you distinguish any physical differences between the in breath and the outbreath?
◆ Do you find that it is possible to make that connection between the breath and your thoughts, physical sensations and emotional experience?

Chapter Summary

◆ The breath has many physiological, neurological and psychological aspects to it
◆ Manipulation of the breath can cause changes in these factors to help engender different states of mind, feelings and bodily experiences
◆ A range of common factors for all psychotherapeutic approaches can all be influenced by meditation
◆ A foundational meditation technique using the breath as the object of attention can be practised to bring about a general therapeutic stance incorporating these common factors

◆ There are specific techniques to be used to establish the meditation frame, which is common to all the meditation techniques in the book

◆ By becoming familiar with the breath, you can create a *home* in the breath that allows you to access this mindset more readily.

References

Alper, S.A. (2016). *Mindfulness Meditation in Psychotherapy*. California, CA: New Harbinger Publications.

Balban, M.Y., Neri, E., Kogon, M.M., Weed, L., Nouriani, B., Jo, B., Holl, G., Zeitzer, J.M., Spiegel, D. and Huberman, A.D. (2023). Brief structured respiration practices enhance mood and reduce physiological arousal. *Cell Reports Medicine*, 4, 100895, pp.01–10.

Ben-Tal, A., Shamailov, S.S. and Paton, J.F.R. (2012). Evaluating the physiological significance of respiratory sinus arrhythmia: Looking beyond ventilation-perfusion efficiency. *The Journal of Physiology*, 590(8), pp.1989–2008.

Bernardi, L., Spadacini, G., Bellwon, J., Hajric, R., Roskamm, H. and Frey, A.W. (1998). Effect of breathing rate on oxygen saturation and exercise performance in chronic heart failure. *Lancet*, 351(9112), pp.1308–1311.

Bion, W.R. (1962). *Learning from Experience*. London: Heinemann.

Bremer, B., Wu, Q., Mora Álvarez, M.G., Hölzel, B.K., Wilhelm, M., Hell, E., Tavacioglu, E.E., Torske, A. and Koch, K. (2022). Mindfulness meditation increases default mode, salience, and central executive network connectivity. *Scientific Reports*, 12(1), p.13219.

Burgess, J., Ekanayake, B., Lowe, A., Dunt, D., Thien, F. and Dharmage, S.C. (2011). Systematic review of the effectiveness of breathing retraining in asthma management. *Expert Review of Respiratory Medicine*, 5(6), pp.789–807.

Byeon, K., Choi, J.-O., Yang, J.H., Sung, J., Park, S.W., Oh, J.K. and Hong, K.P. (2012). The response of the vena cava to abdominal breathing. *Journal of Alternative and Complementary Medicine*, 18(2), pp.153–157.

Castonguay, L.G. and Beutler, L.E. (2006). *Principles of Therapeutic Change that Work*. New York: Oxford University Press.

Condon, P., Desbordes, G., Miller, W.B. and DeSteno, D. (2013). Meditation increases compassionate responses to suffering. *Psychological Science*, 24(10), pp.2125–2127.

Del Negro, C.A., Funk, G.D. and Feldman, J.L. (2018). Breathing matters. *Nature Reviews Neuroscience*, 19(6), pp.351–367.

Fox, K.C.R., Zakarauskas, P., Dixon, M., Ellamil, M., Thompson, E. and Christoff, K. (2012). Meditation experience predicts introspective accuracy. *PLoS ONE*, 7(9), p.e45370.

Goenka, S.N. (1987). *The Discourse Summaries*. Maharashtra: Vipassana Research Institute.

Hofmann, S.G., Grossman, P. and Hinton, D.E. (2011). Loving-kindness and compassion meditation: Potential for psychological interventions. *Clinical Psychology Review*, 31(7), pp.1126–1132.

Ito, S., Sasano, H., Sasano, N., Hayano, J., Fisher, J.A. and Katsuya, H. (2006). Vagal nerve activity contributes to improve the efficiency of pulmonary gas exchange in hypoxic humans. *Experimental Physiology*, 91(5), pp.935–941.

Jha, A.P., Krompinger, J. and Baime, M.J. (2007). Mindfulness training modifies subsystems of attention. *Cognitive, Affective, & Behavioral Neuroscience*, 7(2), pp.109–119.

Kuppusamy, M., Dilara, K., Ravishankar, P. and Julius, A. (2017). Effect of Bhrāmarī Prāṇāyāma practice on pulmonary function in healthy adolescents: A randomized control study. *Ancient Science of Life*, 36(4), p.196.

Li, C., Chang, Q., Zhang, J. and Chai, W. (2018). Effects of slow breathing rate on heart rate variability and arterial baroreflex sensitivity in essential hypertension. *Medicine*, 97(18), p.e0639.

Livesley, W.J. (2007). An integrated approach to the treatment of personality disorder. *Journal of Mental Health*, 16(1), pp.131–148.

Loizzo, J.J. (2016). The subtle body: An interoceptive map of central nervous system function and meditative mind-brain-body integration. *Annals of the New York Academy of Sciences*, 1373(1), pp.78–95.

Lundberg, J.O. (2008). Nitric oxide and the paranasal sinuses. *The Anatomical Record: Advances in Integrative Anatomy and Evolutionary Biology*, 291(11), pp.1479–1484.

Lutz, A., Brefczynski-Lewis, J., Johnstone, T. and Davidson, R.J. (2008). Regulation of the neural circuitry of emotion by compassion meditation: Effects of meditative expertise. *PLoS ONE*, 3(3), p.e1897.

Lutz, A., Greischar, L.L., Perlman, D.M. and Davidson, R.J. (2009). BOLD signal in insula is differentially related to cardiac function during compassion meditation in experts vs. novices. *NeuroImage*, 47(3), pp.1038–1046.

MacLean, K.A., Ferrer, E., Aichele, S.R., Bridwell, D.A., Zanesco, A.P., Jacobs, T.L., King, B.G., Rosenberg, E.L., Sahdra, B.K., Shaver, P.R., Wallace, B.A., Mangun, G.R. and Saron, C.D. (2010). Intensive meditation training improves perceptual discrimination and sustained attention. *Psychological Science*, 21(6), pp.829–839.

Mahasi, S. (2016). *Manual of Insight*. Massachusetts: Wisdom Publications.

McCollum, E.E. (2014). *Mindfulness for Therapists: Practice for the Heart*. New York: Routledge.

Nestor, J. (2022). *Breath: The New Science of a Lost Art*. Riverhead Books.

Norcross, J.C. (Ed.). (2011). *Psychotherapy Relationships that Work: Evidence-Based Responsiveness*, 2nd Edition. New York: Oxford University Press.

Ochs, M., Nyengaard, J.R., Jung, A., Knudsen, L., Voigt, M., Wahlers, T., Richter, J. and Gundersen, H.J.G. (2004). The number of alveoli in the human lung. *American Journal of Respiratory and Critical Care Medicine*, 169(1), pp.120–124.

Pace, T.W.W., Negi, L.T., Adame, D.D., Cole, S.P., Sivilli, T.I., Brown, T.D., Issa, M.J. and Raison, C.L. (2009). Effect of compassion meditation on neuroendocrine, innate immune and behavioral responses to psychosocial stress. *Psychoneuroendocrinology*, 34(1), pp.87–98.

Perl, O., Ravia, A., Rubinson, M., Eisen, A., Soroka, T., Mor, N., Secundo, L. and Sobel, N. (2019). Human non-olfactory cognition phase-locked with inhalation. *Nature Human Behaviour*, 3(5), pp.501–512.

Pramanik, T., Pudasaini, B. and Prajapati, R. (2010). Immediate effect of a slow pace breathing exercise Bhramari Pranayama on blood pressure and heart rate. *Nepal Medical College Journal*, 12(3), pp.154–157.

Siegel, D.J. (2010). *The Mindful Therapist: A Clinician's Guide to Mindsight and Neural Integration*. New York: W.W. Norton & Co.

Stromberg, S.E., Russell, M.E. and Carlson, C.R. (2015). Diaphragmatic breathing and its effectiveness for the management of motion sickness. *Aerospace Medicine and Human Performance*, 86(5), pp.452–457.

Tang, Y.-Y., Hölzel, B.K. and Posner, M.I. (2015). The neuroscience of mindfulness meditation. *Nature Reviews Neuroscience*, 16(4), pp.213–225.

Trivedi, G.Y., Sharma, K., Banshi Saboo, S., Kathirvel, A., Konat, V., Zapadia, Prajapati, P.J., Benani, U., Patel, K. and Shah, S. (2023). Humming (simple Bhramari Pranayama) as a stress buster: A Holter-based study to analyze heart rate variability (HRV) parameters during Bhramari, physical activity, emotional stress, and sleep. *Cureus*, 15(4), e37527.

Vialatte, F.B., Bakardjian, H., Prasad, R. and Cichocki, A. (2009). EEG paroxysmal gamma waves during Bhramari Pranayama: A yoga breathing technique. *Consciousness and Cognition*, 18(4), pp.977–988.

Vlemincx, E., Van Diest, I. and Van den Bergh, O. (2016). A sigh of relief or a sigh to relieve: The psychological and physiological relief effect of deep breaths. *Physiology & Behavior*, 165, pp.127–135.

Vostatek, P., Novák, D., Rychnovský, T. and Rychnovská, Š (2013). Diaphragm postural function analysis using magnetic resonance imaging. *PLoS ONE*, 8(3), p.e56724.

Weitzberg, E. and Lundberg, J.O.N. (2002). Humming greatly increases nasal nitric oxide. *American Journal of Respiratory and Critical Care Medicine*, 166(2), pp.144–145.

Winnicott, D.W. (1960). The theory of the parent-infant relationship. *The International Journal of Psycho-Analysis*, 41, pp.585–595.

Zaccaro, A., Piarulli, A., Laurino, M., Garbella, E., Menicucci, D., Neri, B. and Gemignani, A. (2018). How breath-control can change your life: A systematic review on psycho-physiological correlates of slow breathing. *Frontiers in Human Neuroscience*, 12(353), pp.01–16.

Zelano, C., Jiang, H., Zhou, G., Arora, N., Schuele, S., Rosenow, J. and Gottfried, J.A. (2016). Nasal respiration entrains human limbic oscillations and modulates cognitive function. *The Journal of Neuroscience*, 36(49), pp.12448–12467.

3 The Psychoanalytic Stance
External Listening

I have divided these two sections on the psychoanalytic stance into two themes based on what Parsons (2007) calls internal and external analytic listening. Internal listening is the capacity to observe those reactions that arise within the therapist's mind and body and external listening more observing the client's words, affect and body. Therefore, internal listening will be based on Sigmund Freud's concept of evenly suspended attention and Wilfred Bion's idea of working *without memory or desire* and negative capability. External listening will be associated with Paula Heimann and Heinrich Racker's approaches of using the therapist's countertransference as a way of understanding the client, as well as Bion and the post-Bionians – Thomas Ogden, the da Rocha Barros' (Elizabeth and Elias) and Antonino Ferro's use of the concepts of the therapist's reveries. Guided meditation techniques will be offered that have been extrapolated from how these theories and practices map onto the meditation framework.

Evenly Suspended Attention

Sigmund Freud (1856–1939) was an Austrian neurologist and founder of psychoanalysis – the clinical method of treating and assessing psychopathology through dialogue between therapist and client, as well as a theory to understand the mind and behaviour emerging from it. He was and continues to be an

DOI: 10.4324/9781003382959-3

influential and controversial figure in the fields of psychology, psychiatry and neurology, even as the various schools of psychoanalysis have developed significantly since his lifetime. While I have framed this section as the psychoanalytic stance around Freud's idea of evenly suspended attention, I think this section and the following, on Bion's concept of *without memory or desire* and negative capability, also apply as general stances from which therapists from many modalities operate. As such, I think it offers a good starting point for understanding how meditation can serve to support the development of a particular state of mind which a therapist might occupy in the consultation room. I hope from the meditation described in the previous chapter, there is an idea forming about how the breath can be used to change the experience of the mind and body, the latter part of the meditation being where we could experiment and explore how these aspects interact a bit more. I will now take this concept and practice to focus on a particular therapeutic mindset.

> The technique, however, is a very simple one. As we shall see, it rejects the use of any special expedient (even that of taking notes). It consists simply in not directing one's notice to anything in particular and in maintaining the same 'evenly suspended attention'.
>
> (Freud, 1912, p. 111)

Freud posed this specific style of attention as a means to manage the large amount of client information coming in. Rather than attempting to process and recall everything the client has said, the therapist should listen to the manner in which the client speaks, rather focussing so much on the content. Albeit aspirational instead of set in stone, this is not a memory exercise or a method to process data, but rather a means to gain insight into the client's unconscious by the therapist using their own unconscious as a tool of reflection. In the spirit of this, it has also been proposed that a more accurate translation from Freud's German might be evenly swaying attention (Hoffer, 2020). Be it evenly swaying, free-floating or hovering, I think all sum up this idea that the attention is dynamic and not entirely fixed on one point which can be reflected in a meditation that is more open than focussed on the concentration range.

> The doctor should be opaque to his clients and, like a mirror, should show them nothing but what is shown to him.
>
> (Freud, 1912, p. 118)

> … the doctor's unconscious is able, from the derivatives of the unconscious which are communicated to him, to reconstruct that unconscious which has determined the client's free associations.
>
> (Freud, 1912, p. 116)

> … the attitude which the analytic physician could most advantageously adopt was to surrender himself to his own unconscious mental activity, in a state of evenly suspended attention, to avoid so far as possible reflection and the construction of conscious expectations, not to try to fix anything that he heard particularly in his memory, and by these means to catch the drift of the client's unconscious with his own unconscious.
>
> (Freud, 1923, p. 235)

This is the therapist's mind as an extension of the client's unconscious and their free associations, the thoughts that bubble up from the unconscious in a spontaneous way connected with what had just occurred, albeit not necessarily logically, as the conduit. The therapist does not bring their own issues. Freud implored therapists to undergo their own therapy so as not to react to their own personal issues (for him, this kind of counter-transference was an obstruction and continues to be thought so by many therapists) and stick to what the client is bringing to the session. Therefore, undergoing therapy is a central part of any psychotherapy training. This reduces any resistance to the process of receiving the client's unconscious communications and increases the therapist's capacity to manage the impact of being a therapist. Likewise, I will show how a well-developed meditation practice can support the therapist in the development of this ability to stick closely with the client and become more receptive to their communication.

First, the nature of the mental qualities required for this evenly suspended attention must be interrogated. The therapist is not to be drawn into the client's experience but rather sits outside and acts as an independent mediator. This is achieved with the quality of abstinence. The ability to tolerate abstinence can be challenging and the urge to speak or act out can be great. This is, of course, how silence can bring a client to speak more, but also that they can find silence quite persecutory, so a balance between silence and managing a client's anxiety is key. Meditation can help to develop this mental quality whereby an abstinent stance can be tolerated with time to think and make more meaningful and well-timed interventions. This occurs in the process of meditating, whereby noticing the mind deviating from its focus and returning it, the function of mindfulness, can help develop the necessary patience and tolerance of frustration when the mind might not be doing what we would like. Equally, by not talking in meditation, one becomes more comfortable with sitting in silence and one's inner world becomes less chaotic reducing the urge to distract from those inner thoughts and experiences with speech or action. Therefore, there is less necessity to manage silence by filling it with thoughts, speech or action. Some of that space initially can also be filled with awareness of the breath and sometimes turning attention to the breath in the consultation room can be very beneficial. Eventually, the raw experience can be tolerated without too much discomfort, evasion or action.

Freud did not expect the therapist to choose what they listened to from the client. Of course, that is not limited to the content of the client's speech but also the unconscious clues included in parapraxes (slips of the tongue), dreams and the transference. There is a contemporaneous analysis of defences and interpretations of transference and resistance. The attention must float, suspend or hover between these current issues and also make references to childhood situations or other relationships. With all these issues, the therapist should not become too focussed on any of them especially, but pay more attention to the client's free associative flow. Therefore, there is a strong focus on the client, but also the therapist allows their own experience to unfold in their mind as a proxy to understand the client.

There is a balance to be had between making interventions and listening to the client. The therapist must discern whether an interpretation is useful and if it serves the client or the therapist's interest to come across as someone who can show they know or empathise. To judge whether saying something might be too overwhelming for the client at that time, or if the therapist is holding back for fear of stirring something up that could be too challenging for the therapist to contain. At the same time, it could be most beneficial to listen in an active way and to provide that holding environment for the client to be able to express their thoughts and feelings no matter how disturbing they could appear. As a former supervisor, Katrina Wynne used to express, borrowing terminology from medical prescriptions, *it is a matter of timing and dosage*. This balance between abstaining and intervening is one of particular familiarity to a meditator.

There is an equilibrium to be had between the ardency and effort in meditation to actively take up skilful and abandon unskilful mental qualities, but at the same time not holding the mind too focussed or fixed so as to allow for the experience to unfold. There is the doing – perhaps breathing in a particular way, but also letting go of certain aspects such as mind wandering. This is equivalent to the therapist abstaining and allowing the client to open up or interpreting and actively doing. The therapist's mind is therefore focussed and alert to what, but more how, the client is speaking in the present moment. They are waiting to see what comes up in their own mind as an extension of the client's unconscious in an ardent manner, evaluating which of these thoughts might be most skilful to use as interpretations or whether abstaining may be more helpful. Meditation, especially in the particular way suggested below, helps with the development of all these mental qualities.

The technique continues after the *establishing the meditation frame* exercise to establish evenly suspended attention by taking the attention to follow the breath as it comes in and goes with a more open awareness of the breath instead of being so focussed on a point. The breath is allowed to settle as is rather than adjusting it as we have done in the first meditation. The breath is now the equivalent of the client's voice and presence in the consultation room and concentrating on it focusses on awareness as alertness in the present moment to increase the focus of concentration. When thoughts, perceptions, fantasies arise, the attention is brought back to the breath. This act of remembering to keep the breath in mind helps develop the faculty of mindfulness. By continuing to bring attention back to the breath, ardency is used to refrain from being drawn away from the object of attention helping to develop the analytic attitude and skill of abstinence.

Often, the mind will head off in one direction or another, but with careful training, the capacity to keep the attention on the object to improve mindfulness and alertness can be developed. This is, of course, an invaluable skill when working as a therapist with clients. The aim, however, is not to empty the mind of thoughts and to stay in the present moment, this would make the mind too focussed and not in a space where there could be an interpersonal experience. Rather, the evenly suspended aspect is to remain focussed enough on the breath but open enough to allow thoughts to arise and the attention to shift between objects.

This technique is closer to focussed awareness on the concentration range, as it is more focussed around a point of the breath (albeit not too focussed as expressed above). It also leans towards non-judgemental awareness on the discernment range as the object (the breath in the meditation and the client with the unconscious communications arising in the consulting room) is not judged to be skilful or unskilful. The factor of mindfulness takes the most active part of the technique, so it is most predominant in the range. However, the floating and suspended nature of the awareness means mindfulness, alertness and ardency are all employed.

After establishing the meditation frame as in the first meditation exercise and developed a sensitivity to the breath as well as using it to develop a certain level-headedness and focus, we will use the breath to help establish this faculty of external listening. While some part of the meditation requires allowing the breath to remain as it is, I recognise that when the mind moves significantly away from the task at hand, it might be helpful to adjust the breath, just as we did in the first exercise, to bring the attention back – be that with a few sighs, some slower breaths or more rough breaths depending on what works for you. However, the breath will eventually be allowed to settle, with the meditation activity itself establishing the particular mindset of free-floating and even suspension, remaining fairly open after the initial focus *simply in not directing one's notice to anything in particular* as Freud (1912, p. 111) described.

While evenly suspended attention is a mindset that I'm sure resonates with therapists who practice in different modalities, not just psychodynamic, it can be one that is paired with the open-ended and increased frequency of psychoanalytic work. Many therapists work with more brief models, including short-term psychodynamic work, whereby there isn't the time to allow for the unfolding and emerging themes to arise. Therefore, a more focussed and evaluative mindset may be more fitting. This issue of time and the requirement for a different internal setting is expressed by Gertrud Mander in her book on brief psycho-dynamic approaches (2000) where the emphasis on focus and evaluation as selective neglect is emphasised:

> Theirs is a craft of quick decisions, of no second chances, of striking the iron while it is hot and of ruthlessly pur-suing an avenue once it has been chosen. There is no time for regrets at missed opportunities. Like their more passive and leisurely colleagues, brief therapists always work on several levels at once, processing and responding to the patient's communications while sim-ultaneously monitoring the transference and counter-transference constellation and the diagnostic hypothesis. However, in contrast to the passive analytic colleagues practising evenly hovering attention, they endeavour to stay on focus at all times, to exercise selective attention and selective neglect and to steer the therapeutic pro-cess briskly along a route that involves no hesitation or resting place. There is a clear purpose to every interven-tion, which will be linked to the chosen focus and to the

known and anticipated ending of the therapy, and all of this serves to push the process as fast and as far as possible in the chosen direction. At the same time, there will be a constant close observation of the patient's ego functioning, as any sign of a regression to dependence needs to be recognized and if possible to be nipped in the bud, as will sidetracking manoeuvres on the part of the patient like being offered dreams, memories or new problems not directly relating to the focus.

(Mander, 2000, p. 61)

Therefore, while occupying a similar even suspension, there is an increase in focus compared with a more open state of concentration and more evaluating opposed to non-judgemental discernment. We can translate this to meditation technique, when considering the breath meditation method illustrated below. In the meditation method, it therefore might be necessary to have an increase in focus by selecting a smaller aspect of the breath, such as the tip of the nose or movement of the abdomen, instead of the full length of the breath. Likewise, a more evaluating mindset can be engendered by bringing the attention back to the breath more firmly, occupying a position with more alertness and making that discernment between where you might want your attention or not, this being a function of ardency.

Thinking on the other end of the concentration spectrum to this approach with brief psychotherapy – Patrick Casement, a British psychoanalyst, brings in an idea of *unfocussed listening*. This mindset would be one that has a more open awareness than evenly suspended attention and brings more space into the therapeutic relationships in stark contrast to the description of brief psychotherapy above:

I regard this as a first step beyond that of the familiar "evenly suspended attention," with which analysts are encouraged to listen to the overall drift of a patient's communications. When I think that I am beginning to understand what is being communicated in a session, I find that it helps me to avoid preconceived ideas about this if I first abstract the recognizable themes from what a patient is saying, and hold these provisionally away from the overt context. Also, if I sometimes listen to the identified themes with unconscious symmetry in mind, it helps to show up the different possible meanings that can then emerge. For instance, if a patient were to say "My boss is angry with me," this can be silently abstracted as "someone is angry with someone." Whose anger with whom then remains unclear, and this can be considered with a more open mind than otherwise would be possible. It could be a statement of fact, objectively reported; it could be a reference to the patient's anger, projected onto the boss; it could be a displaced reference to the transference, the therapist seen as angry; or it could be an oblique reference to the patient being angry with the therapist. In practice, this balancing of different potential meanings needs to be integrated into the normal process of internal supervision.

(Casement, 1985, p. 38)

Casement describes how unfocussed listening helps to open up the mind to *internal supervision*:

… a learned but ultimately semi-automatic preconscious process by which the analyst constantly scans behaviors and verbalizations from the point of view of how these might be experienced by the patient, in light of the patient's history and character, and quite apart from how they were formulated and consciously intended by the analyst.

(Casement, 1985, p. xiii)

There is the development of an internal supervisor as an internalising of external supervision and a way for a therapist to work more independently with a client serving:

… to hold the analyst (or therapist) who is learning to hold the patient. This provides the structure of an internal "nursing triad," which can help the therapist to find an inner play-space where the clinical options can be explored (silently or with the patient) rather than remaining blinkered by past thinking that often functions too much like a set of rules.

(Casement, 1985, p. 28)

Therefore, a more open awareness around different aspects of the breath beyond one particular point might be more appropriate with a more non-judgemental attitude to what might be arriving in the mind at any time. This provides the space in the mind for this internal supervisor to develop as well as the mindset of unfocussed listening.

We can therefore map these three approaches onto the range of concentration from focussed to open with the brief psychotherapy approach as the most focussed, evenly suspended attention in the middle and unfocussed listening as having a more open awareness. They also follow along the parameters of discernment with brief psychotherapy as the most evaluating through to unfocussed listening being more non-judgemental. Through the meditation method below, we can establish these different states of mind using the breath as the meditation object and establishing different kinds of concentration and discernment depending on which aspects of the breath the attention is brought to and how it might be decided what is most useful to keep that concentration on. The next section on *Without Memory or Desire and Negative Capability* will bring an even more open, non-judgemental awareness which unfocussed listening may be getting towards.

The following meditation exercise and the others offered throughout this book give examples of how the specific mindsets associated with an assortment of therapeutic approaches can be developed which can occur in a formal way *on the cushion* (as is often expressed to explain the process of sitting in meditation). However, these mindsets can also be brought in before or during sessions with clients. Either that can be a short period of meditation before a session or by using some breaths to establish that same mindset which will have become familiar and associated with the breath from this more formal sitting. This same technique can also be used during a session with a client, while listening to them, or in a silent pause. Just by bringing attention back to the breath, it can help to maintain or re-establish the mind to a specific mindset. These ideas will be explored in more detail in the *In the Consultation Room* section of the *Other Complementary Techniques* chapter.

Meditation Exercise – Developing External Listening, Evenly Suspended Attention

Picking up from having established the meditation frame where we have worked to develop a sense of ease and comfort around a specific area in the breath, we will open up our awareness back to the whole of the body of the breath. Our attention will remain focussed on the breath, noticing the range of sensations that occur throughout the cycle of breathing from the tip of the nose, back of the throat and expansion of the lungs on inhalation followed by the reverse for exhalation. These sensations include the feeling of the movement of air through the body, the temperature of the air in the nose and throat – cooler on breathing in, and warmer on breathing out, the movement of the body most apparent with the chest, shoulders and abdomen and then any other sensations that might be occurring through the shifting of the blood pressure and heart rate throughout the respiratory cycle. There may also be other sensations of warmth, tingling in the peripheries with the blood flow we have discussed before or that we might think about more metaphorically as an effect of the breath's energetic force. There is plenty to notice and observe, the more we look, the more we will find and the act of not interfering or abstinence with the breath will allow the experience to unfold before our attention. Try not to become so fixated on this process that all other experiences are blocked out as we aim for evenly suspended attention with the breath as the object of this mindset. While it might become quite a pleasant experience, that is not the aim of this meditation exercise, as the concentration becomes too focussed and not open enough with too much alertness at play.

Inevitably, the mind will float off to a thought, a more involved fantasy about the past or future concern, or towards some discomfort in the body all coloured with a particular affect. After noticing where the mind's attention has floated off to be that a thought, a fantasy, a sensation or an affect, with mindful attention, we will gently remember the task at hand and bring out awareness back to the breath starting again with the ardency to remain on the breath and notice when being pulled away. When bringing the attention back, try as always to be gentle and kind to yourself as we can all too easily end up finding the process frustrating.

Thus, the attention becomes free-floating, hovering and evenly suspended. The aim is not to stay as fixed as possible but to develop robustness in the face of this movement, increasing comfort to remain focussed, but equally capable of shifting the attention to notice what is happening instead of being thrown about unthinkingly. Each time the mind hovers off, notice where it has gone be that a thought, fantasy, physical sensation or affective experience before floating back to the breath.

If you're becoming so frustrated with this process that it's feeling overwhelming, there are increasingly uncomfortable physical sensations that are intolerable or the amount of time that it is possible to stay with the breath is a matter of only a couple of seconds, then it might be necessary to be spending more time establishing the meditation frame and settling the mind. Alternatively, we can bring some of the techniques to use the breath to settle the mind if agitated, or increase stimulation if drowsy by altering the manner of breathing. This can help to manage some of the discomforts before returning to the process of developing this evenly suspended attention within the meditation. Equally, the process of noticing where the mind has gone and approaching it with a non-judgemental attitude of discernment can help to reduce all three of these experiences through the development of a more abstinent, neutral and robust mindset that can tolerate more of this free-floating. Sometimes, we can notice how we have a desire for a particular mindset in meditation – usually wanting no thoughts or some kind of pleasant physical sensation, to stay with the breath for longer, for the meditation timer to finish and many other wishes. In the same way, by noticing frustrations with a neutral, non-judgemental stance rather than fighting them, their power over us is reduced and they will slowly become less burdensome. Hoping for a given outcome ends up putting the cart before the horse and will likely provoke the very mindset that had been not wanted.

We can consider the different mindsets for brief psychotherapy – more focussed and evaluating and unfocussed listening – a more open and non-judgemental awareness. For a brief psychotherapy mindset, focus on one particular area of the breath and quickly return to that area whenever you notice your mind wandering, try to breathe in a way that engenders higher levels of alertness, allowing you to stay with the breath. For an approach closer to unfocussed listening, open up your awareness to the full experience of the breath within the airways and beyond into the limbs, allowing the breath to settle in whichever way it finds itself. Notice where the mind goes, and once it feels ready, bring the attention back to the breath again. Mindfully return to the breath without making judgements about what might be a useful way to breathe or on the content of the mind wandering, rather noting the content.

Having continued with this exercise of following the breath, noticing the movements of the mind and body for the allocated time of the meditation, open your eyes and spend a few minutes reviewing the session.

Some questions on which to reflect:

◆ Can you see how the mind was suspended, hovering or freely floating between positions?
◆ Was it possible to use some of those breathing techniques from the earlier meditation when needed?
◆ How do you feel compared to the start of the meditation?
◆ If thinking about the range of concentration and discernment, were you able to distinguish between those different facets of attention?

Without Memory or Desire and Negative Capability

We have already met Wilfred Bion when thinking about his concept of the therapist in their containing role. In this section, we will look at negative capability and his perspective on the mindset of the psychotherapist as templates on which to map meditation techniques. While evenly suspended attention and Bion's instructions from his infamous paper *Notes on Memory and Desire* are often bracketed together as instructions on the type of attention psychodynamically inclined therapists are to employ, there are some differences which I will elaborate on here, before reflecting on how this type of attention can be engendered by a specific meditation technique.

Bion instructed the therapist to:

Obey the following rules:

1. Memory: Do not remember past sessions. The greater the impulse to remember what has been said or done, the more the need to resist it. This impulse can present itself as a wish to remember something that has happened because it appears to have precipitated an emotional crisis: no crisis should be allowed to breach this rule. The supposed events must not be allowed to occupy the mind. Otherwise the evolution of the session will not be observed at the only time when it can be observed – while it is taking place.
2. Desires: The psychoanalyst can start by avoiding any desires for the approaching end of the session (or week, or term). Desires for results, 'cure' or even understanding must not be allowed to proliferate.

These rules must be obeyed all the time and not simply during the sessions. In time the psychoanalyst will become more aware of the pressure of memories and desires and more skilled at eschewing them.

(Bion, 1967, pp. 273–274)

According to Bion, the human mind has a natural tendency to remember past experiences and desires, which can often interfere with our ability to experience the present moment fully. He believed that this tendency could be especially problematic in therapy, as individuals may become preoccupied with their past experiences and desires. This releases the therapist from the therapy, becoming an exercise in history taking, which was Freud's intent with evenly suspended attention. In addition to this was Bion's vision of the process of psychoanalysis occurring in the here and now between therapist and client on an unconscious and emotional level rather than a more factual and analytical level.

> In every consulting-room, there ought to be two rather frightened people: the client and the psychoanalyst. If they are not both frightened, one wonders why they are bothering to find out what everyone knows.
>
> (Bion, 1990, p. 5)

The quote brings to mind the metaphor of being *in the trenches together*. As a First World War veteran, being in the trenches (or being in a tank regiment alongside them) was a formative experience for a young Bion. Bion developed the concept of *without memory or desire* that overcomes the tendency to reach for historical facts and to intellectualise the therapeutic experience which might avoid the more raw, challenging and frightening emotional experiences of being an effective therapist. This concept refers to a mental state in which an individual is fully present in the moment, free from the influence of these past experiences and desires. In this state, therapists are able to fully engage with their thoughts and emotions in the present moment without being held back by what may have happened before in the therapy, the client's history or focussing on a goal-orientated process.

> I mean Negative Capability, that is, when a man is capable of being in uncertainties, mysteries, doubts, without any irritable reaching after fact and reason.
>
> (Keats, 1899, p. 277)

This refers to the ability to tolerate ambiguity, ambiguity, and not-knowing in the therapeutic process. It is the capacity to remain open and receptive to new ideas, experiences, and emotions without prematurely imposing preconceptions or theories onto them. The term negative capability was originally coined by the poet John Keats to describe the qualities of embracing equivocality and contradictions without attempting to resolve them too quickly. Bion adopted this term to describe where the therapist's ability to tolerate the unknown and the inexplicable is critical in helping clients explore their unconscious. According to Bion, the psychoanalytic process requires the therapist to avoid premature interpretations and allow the client's unconscious thoughts and emotions to emerge without interference. Therapists can therefore, help clients gain deeper insights into their inner selves and overcome psychological obstacles. Therapists must be comfortable with the limits of their own knowledge and recognise that the therapeutic process involves a certain degree of unpredictability and uncertainty. This can be arrived at by the therapist embodying this attitude within themselves. We can see how the attitudes of negative capability and those *without memory or desire* both point towards a similar approach.

Looking at these mindsets through the lens of the meditation framework, they have an open as opposed to focussed awareness. We are trying to take in the breadth of experience in the here and now with a non-judgemental attitude in terms of discernment, for we are not favouring one set of experiences over another. To reach this point, alertness is the most predominate quality that we aim for due to a focus on the present, but we employ mindfulness to remember to stay there when the mind wanders. There is less emphasis on ardency – trying to take up or drop certain characteristics to support the non-judgemental attitude. The mind remains relaxed, not to be drawn away, through a non-resistance opposed to effort. Through this non-resistance there grows a capacity to tolerate more challenging mindsets not through action but a robustness, comfort with ambiguity and leaning towards thinking and feeling instead of action. We can contrast this with the description of evenly suspended attention above and how this employs a less focussed, more open awareness, both sharing a non-judgemental attitude, perhaps more so here and also alertness being more predominate. The description of the mindset brought to brief psychotherapy from that same chapter employs a state with even more focus and evaluating discernment with unfocussed listening being closer to this chapter.

As the title of the very first meditation book I read from the Zen Buddhist tradition puts it, we are *Opening the Hand of Thought* (Uchiyama, 2004). *Without memory or desire* is the state of mind whereby we are not clinging, grasping or chasing after a particular state of mind or possession. The mind is relaxed, open and unencumbered by the stresses associated with regrets from the past and wishes for the future. For those familiar with the concept of *just sitting* in the practice of Zen Buddhism known as *Shikantaza*, it is a state of allowing experiences to unfold in the present moment in a heightened state of alertness, watchful of the flow of experiences within the mind. There is evidence that Bion was aware of Zen Buddhism (Zhang, 2019) so I can see how the similarities may have evolved together for him. The first part of this meditation method is the section which is probably also most in line with the present moment, choiceless, non-judgemental awareness that secular mindfulness approaches often employ. We see this clinically most of all in mindfulness-based therapies such as MBCT and MBSR in which readers may be trained.

Meditation Exercise – Developing External Listening, Without Memory or Desire and Negative Capability

For this meditation, we will spend a bit more time in the establishing the frame meditation method. After having taken the meditation posture, a short survey of the body and how it feels, we will remain on the part where we notice the content of the mind and emotional landscape before putting aside the thoughts and feelings that might be at the forefront of our minds. See if you can notice where the mind wanders in terms of concerns about the past or worries about what might be coming up in the body or with affect. Try initially to put them aside until it gets to the point where things might become repetitive and the same thoughts or feelings are coming up. By staying with this part of the meditation for a bit longer, it will have the effect of helping us to stay in this mode of negative capability. At this point, we return to establishing the meditation frame setting the intention to sit for the period on the timer and take the three sighs with which all our meditations begin and establishing the frame by using the breath as the subject of attention.

Part 1 – Embracing Uncertainties

In order to set the open awareness and non-judgemental aspect of this meditation, we will move on from focussing on the breath and allow our awareness to settle in an open way – not focussing on anything in particular. When something does arise in the mind be that a sensation, a thought, a feeling or a fantasy we will notice it rather than dive into it, in a sense, have one part of the mind watching another. Now, this can be a challenging state of mind to stay in as all sorts of difficult and uncomfortable experiences can arise, though not always, I don't wish to cast this meditation as a necessarily painful one. Often, the mind will draw us towards an alluring fantasy, such as a future holiday or any other exciting or tempting possibility. At other times, we may become immersed in a comfortable physical sensation such as a tingling feeling on the skin or warmth in the chest. The key is to try and keep our attention in a more separate, detached perspective and allow these experiences to arise and pass away observing this as a reality to which we aren't completely attached and at the mercy of being thrown around by. To develop a state of negative capability, we remain in a place without expectation or reaching for a certain experience while also tolerating the uncertainty of being in a place which might be quite ambiguous in nature.

At points, it might be too challenging. If the mind is too unsettled and it is too difficult to maintain this position of negative capability, then spend some time back with the breath adjusting the breathing to bring about some ease and comfort in the mind and body before returning to this mindset just described. The aim of this and other meditations isn't to have a pleasant experience, one can get lost in both these feelings and the desire to re-experience and intensify it. However, the relief and solace that can be found there can provide an incentive to continue meditating and a firm foundation from which other mindsets can then grow.

Perhaps you find it possible to get here, perhaps not. Try not to get too frustrated with yourself as this will then create another layer of judgement on top of the initial cause for frustration. Embrace the paradox of putting effort into allowing a spontaneous event to unfurl. This is a state of play. Let the experience unfold without judgement as to whether it is good or bad, pleasant or unpleasant, desirable or undesirable and without following the experiences too much. Let them pass by like the clouds in the sky. Think of yourself as occupying the position of the sky observing and noticing the clouds, sun, moon, stars rain, rain or snow as the different sensations, thoughts, feelings and fantasies. You are aware of them, you are not interfering with them, you are allowing them to drift into view in whatever form they are before they float away leaving no trace of regret, guilt or sadness. Sometimes the wind is strong and the clouds or rain move quickly, sometimes the days are longer and the sun rises and sets more quickly, other times slowly. Either way, all these phenomena arise and then disappear, and the sky remains there. This is the mindset of no memory or desire with the quality of negative capability.

Having remained in this position for some time, and if feeling ready, we can take this mindset of negative capability and by using a process of self-enquiry bring about the frame of mind from a different point of view. It is up to the meditator, perhaps this first method is sufficient for them, sometimes having another technique can complement and enrich the experience

Part 2 – Self-Enquiry

We will do this by consciously asking ourselves questions and then seeing what experiences arise. We can think of the questions as a kind of mantra, refrain or repetitive phrase to stimulate a certain part of our minds. It can be a helpful hook to keep the mind more on track as well as open up for more creative possibilities. Try repeating the following in your mind (or if helpful vocally):

♦ What is happening right now?
♦ How is it feeling right now?

This enquiry can help to cut off any arising experiences from becoming too absorbing and helps to maintain the state of alertness which at times might become too demanding. It can help to stimulate this state of negative capability. We can shift between this technique and the previous depending on what allows the mind to settle into a position without memory or desire. Perhaps a different phrase spontaneously comes into your mind and if you feel that could offer a more meaningful mantra then stay with that. It can help to repeat the questions slowly, almost without registering the meaning consciously. There is not necessarily a need to answer the questions, but rather, the aim is to see what experiences arise from them.

After practising one or both of these two techniques, there may be a sense that behind the mental and bodily experiences arising, a mindset of negative capability is present which allows for a calmer and more settled meditation but also a different attitude with less of a judgemental state of mind and a greater ability to tolerate the uncertainty that can arise especially when working as a therapist.

When you have completed the meditation, open your eyes and spend a few minutes reviewing the session. Some questions on which to reflect:

♦ How was it settling the mind down initially and establishing the sense of open, non-judgemental awareness with a focus on alertness?
♦ Did you find it possible to get to the point of something akin to negative capability with reference to your breath and the experiences that were coming up?
♦ What arose from the self-enquiry that you tried, did they allow for this mindset to become more accessible?
♦ What was most challenging and what might be useful for next time?

Chapter Summary

♦ Freud's concept of evenly suspended attention offers a particular perspective on psychoanalytic external listening which can be developed with breath meditation

♦ Brief psychotherapy and unfocused listening offer perspectives on either end of the concentration spectrum (focused and open, respectively) with alterations that can be made in the meditation technique to develop these mindsets

♦ Without memory or desire and negative capability are other approaches to external listening with different meditation techniques helping to develop these mindsets

♦ This involves a technique open to more experiences beyond the breath followed by process of self-enquiry.

References

Bion, W.R. (1967). Notes on memory and desire. *Psychoanalytic Forum*, 2, pp.272–273, 279–280.

Bion, W.R. (1990). *Brazilian Lectures: 1973, Sao Paulo; 1974, Rio de Janeiro/ Sao Paulo*. London: Routledge.

Casement, P. (1985). *On Learning from the Patient*. London: Tavistock/ Routledge.

Freud, S. (1912) Recommendations to physicians practising psycho-analysis. In: J. Strachey (Trans & Ed.) *Standard Edition of the Complete Psychological Works of Sigmund Freud*, (vol. 12, 109–120). London: Hogarth Press. Reprinted (1953–1974).

Freud, S. (1923) Two encyclopaedia articles. In: J. Strachey (Trans & Ed.) *Standard Edition of the Complete Psychological Works of Sigmund Freud* (vol. 18, 233–260). London: Hogarth Press. Reprinted (1953–1974).

Hoffer, A. (2020). Psychoanalysis as a two-person meditation: Free association, meditation and Bion. *The American Journal of Psychoanalysis*, 80(3), pp.331–341.

Keats, J. (1899). *The Complete Poetical Works and Letters of John Keats – Cambridge Edition*. Houghton: Mifflin and Company.

Mander, G. (2000). *A Psychodynamic Approach to Brief Therapy*. London: SAGE.

Parsons, M. (2007). Raiding the inarticulate: The internal analytic setting and listening beyond countertransference. *The International Journal of Psychoanalysis*, 88(6), pp.1441–1456.

Uchiyama, K. (2004). *Opening the Hand of Thought: Foundations of Zen Buddhist Practice*. Boston: Simon and Schuster.

Zhang, Y. (2019). Wilfred Bion's annotations in the way of Zen: An investigation into his practical encounters with Buddhist ideas. *Psychoanalysis and History*, 21(3), pp.331–335.

4 The Psychoanalytic Stance

Internal Listening

Countertransference

In this section, I am defining countertransference as the range of thoughts, feelings, sensations and experiences that arise for the therapist in relation to their client. I will describe more how to categorise them as a means to understand the experiences that will arise during the meditation technique consequentially illustrated. It is common to hear in therapists' circles about how countertransference is an interference to the process of therapy, which once identified, is classed as being part of what the therapist is experiencing and less about how the client may be producing that experience for the therapist. Of course, therapists all bring their own pasts, previous and current relationships and selves to a session, but these countertransferential experiences can give unconscious clues as to what the client is going through.

In a departure from the contemporaneous understanding of countertransference, Paula Heimann, a German psychoanalyst working mostly in London after fleeing Nazi Europe in the mid-20th century wrote:

> I would suggest that the analyst along with this freely working attention needs a freely roused emotional sensibility so as to follow the client's emotional movements and unconscious phantasies. Our basic assumption is that the analyst's unconscious understands that of his

DOI: 10.4324/9781003382959-4

client. This rapport on the deep level comes to the surface in the form of feelings which the analyst notices in response to his client, in his 'counter-transference'. This is the most dynamic way in which his client's voice reaches him. In the comparison of feelings roused in himself with his client's associations and behaviour, the analyst possesses a most valuable means of checking whether he has understood or failed to understand his client.

(Heimann, 1950, p. 81)

Heimann moved away from the previous formulation by Freud of countertransference as an unconscious process arising from the analyst's resistance to helping the client, and as a barrier to being able to listen and understand the client. Countertransference, therefore, can be a crucial tool through utilising internal listening to provide more data for the analyst to comprehend the client's unconscious. It is a conscious and preconscious experience of all the feelings felt towards the client produced through unconscious interactions with the client. The psychoanalyst Heinrich Racker, a Polish-Argentine who worked in Brazil after escaping Nazi Europe, explored the use of counter-transference at the same time as Heimann. Racker expressed that countertransference

... may be the greatest danger and at the same time an important tool for understanding

(Racker, 1957, p. 303)

Given that

our unconscious is a very personal 'receiver' and 'transmitter' and we must reckon with frequent distortions of objective reality.

(Racker, 1957, p. 354)

The importance of one's own therapy is therefore crucial for the therapist to determine if a feeling arises from their own issues or as a result of countertransference from the client. Supervision also offers another perspective and prevents the therapist from potentially acting in on their countertransference, managing these distortions and dangers, which, of course, are present. For this reason, I can understand why some therapists may be deterred by the idea of working with their countertransference in this particular way. For me, it offers a powerful and meaningful way to penetrate the many layers of defences with which clients often present. It also brings the therapist alongside the client through a collaborative emotional experience whereby the therapist and client are both experiencing something together, an intersubjective space created during and within the specific environment of the therapy session. This runs counter to the perspective sometimes experienced or expected by a client of a therapist offering them advice, guidance or strategies or perhaps an expert who can tell them what to do or offer a solution to their difficulties. Working with the countertransference alongside transference also brings the experience even more into the present – a more tangible and immediate encounter for a client – with the therapist and parts of their mind of which they may be unaware, rather than solely focussing on past or contemporary relationships outside of the consultation room.

Another interesting perspective is from Parsons (2007), who further expands on the idea of using countertransference. Up until now, we have thought of countertransference as deriving from the therapist, which may be a hinderance and as a response from the client providing information about their experience. Parsons considers a third position – how countertransference that arises solely from the analyst's own psyche garnered by listening analytically to themselves can be utilised to bring fresh creativity and enhance the capacity of the analyst to benefit the analysis. Parsons describes this in relation to alternating between listening to poems and clients. We will see how meditation can be another conduit for this to arise, which I feel like poetry, is a way to tap into something that might seem ineffable in comparison to more direct internal listening. This will be illustrated by the meditation exercise at the end of this chapter as one part of the mind listening to another.

Bion (1959) described the importance of projective identification operating from client to therapist, who can experience the content of what has been projected, just as Klein (1946) described, between mother and baby. The interpretation of this countertransferential experience being of therapeutic value. Also, the ability to tolerate the countertransference with a kind of psychic robustness (Carpy, 1989) can be of benefit even without interpretation, by bringing about psychic change for the client through a partial acting out by the therapist. This emphasises that the role of the therapist isn't to be some kind of psychic punching bag automaton absorbing everything the client throws at them, but rather a living, breathing and feeling part of the therapeutic process.

Psychic robustness is one of the products of a meditation practice as the mind repeatedly learns to tolerate discomfort arising from staying with the meditation object, but returns to it nonetheless and uses resourcefulness to come up with ways to stay there. By truly experiencing the full effect of the countertransference without acting out on it in more than just a partial way, it can give the client an experience which brings about insight. This partial enactment, which Carpy builds on from Brenman Pick (1985), takes the form of both the chosen subject of interpretation and how it is delivered. The therapeutic aspect is derived from the client observing this process. As will be shown, meditation can help to support a certain robustness which can help balance tolerating the full force of countertransference without being overwhelmed by it, at the same time managing this concept of a partial enactment. This can then allow for the consequential analysis of countertransference as per psychoanalytic technique if the therapist is working in this way.

Research into mirror neurons offers neuroscientific evidence for the transference and countertransference phenomena across cognitive, affective and somatic domains. The use of somatic countertransference and a corresponding meditation technique will be explored in the *Body-Centred Psychotherapy – Somatic Perspectives* chapter of this book. Mirror neurons were first discovered when noticing that areas of a monkey's brain respond when a monkey performs a specific action while recognising a similar action by a human or another monkey (Rizzolatti et al., 1996). This effect has been repeated in human subjects with regards to an audiovisual mirroring system (Pizzamiglio et al., 2005). In essence, the neurons fire when stimulated by the witnessed behaviour of another. More widely, they have been posited as the neural basis for empathy through making inter-subjectivity possible by allowing access into and understanding of others' minds (Iacoboni, 2009). Therefore, they have also been suggested as part of the basis of a wide range of other thera-peutic modalities including Eye Movement Desensitisation and Reprocessing (EMDR) (Piedfort-Marin, 2018) and group psy-chotherapy (Schermer, 2010) amongst others. We can, therefore, think about how this might come into psychoanalytic psycho-therapy and this phenomenon of countertransference. Gallese (2009) suggests that mirror neurons underpin a process known as embodied simulation. The description of projective identifica-tion and consequential countertransferential experience on the part of the therapist represents a prelinguistic more primitive expression of this process.

> It is the intersubjective process of embodied simulation, we propose, that permits the kind of direct, noninferential understanding that constitutes a basis for the therapeutic use of the analyst's countertransference reactions. In short, we are witnessing a central aspect of the shift in contem-porary psychoanalysis from a primarily theory-theory account to one that places increased emphasis on a simula-tion theory account in understanding another's mind.
>
> (Gallese, Eagle and Migone, 2007, p. 165)

It is, of course, exciting to consider how there may be a neuroscientific basis for psychoanalytic theories especially due to the long-running accusations of it not being *evidence based* and non-falsifiable (Popper, 1963) as well as the promise of a physical basis for the ineffable and emotional experience of connection with others. That said, I think it's also important to recognise that this area is disputed with issues taken up about a lack of adequate testing in monkeys and evidence against the direct connections between action understanding and mirror neuron systems functioning (Hickok, 2009). The connection specifically between countertransference and mirror neurons has also been

disputed, which while I think it might not be necessary to completely reject, offers the expectation that more research might
be needed. Vivona (2009) suggested the following assumptions
might have been made, which I think also raises questions about
other connections made between neuroscience and psychological phenomena:

> (1) there is a straightforward correspondence between
> observed brain activity and mental activity; (2) simi-
> larity of localized brain activity across individuals signi-
> fies a shared interpersonal experience; (3) an automatic
> brain mechanism enables direct interpersonal sharing
> of experiences in the absence of inference and language.
> Examination of mirror neuron research findings reveals
> that these assumptions are either untested or question-
> able … The present state of mirror neuron research may
> offer us new hypotheses or metaphors, but does not pro-
> vide empirical validation of the proposed models.
>
> (Vivona, 2009)

So, how might all these theories look with reference to a
meditation practice? When meditating, the mind is denied its
usual stimuli. The mind, therefore, looks for other conduits to
cathect this emotional and mental energy. This can be analogous
to a client arriving in therapy for the first time and faced with
someone who might be more silent than they are used to or perhaps more available to listen rather than fill the time with their
thoughts. That available space which would usually be filled
with physical movement, the other person talking, or another
activity, is then often replaced with the client's anxieties. When
first meditating this can often emerge as a physical pain, just how
physical symptoms arise from mental disturbances. Equally, it
can cause mental discomfort which emerges as a desire to stop
meditating, or the mind being filled with fantasies or daydreams
about all the other things you could be doing rather than this
admittedly unusual activity of sitting quietly.

As a meditator becomes more comfortable in this state of
abstaining and not satisfying the desire to think about other

objects or feeling other sensations, the mind becomes more settled and concentrated. This concentration allows for observation of the mind from a less reactive position and a wider range of more subtle experiences arise including feelings, bodily sensations, thoughts and perceptions. These are the equivalent of the countertransferential experience in the room with the client. However, instead of the object being the client's unconscious or as in the previous meditation techniques described the breath, it is one part of the mind observing another.

Rather than being absorbed by these countertransferential experiences, the part of the mind occupying a specific state of alertness, mindfulness and ardency can take these as their object. This is not a split in a schizoid manner because the specific nature of the meditative internal stance and frame allows for a calmer, less reactive and more objective look – listening analytically to oneself (Parsons, 2007). There needs to be a high level of internal ego strength and mental stability to experience it in this way, or else the initial physical and emotional pain that arises can become too uncomfortable or overwhelming. Therefore, usually a meditation practice is built up over time, starting with shorter sessions lasting just a few minutes.

Indeed, after attending many intensive silent retreats, I have observed some attendees finding the experience overwhelming and have seen and heard anecdotal evidence of even psychotic responses to the demanding nature of this state of mind. Often, at the end of a silent retreat, some attendees are left in a somewhat manic state, talking at a great rate to seemingly evacuate the build-up of mental content over the period of the retreat. It is hoped that most trained therapists have the degree of ego strength required to tolerate these experiences and there is no expectation to jump into an intensive retreat, but rather to slowly build up a regular practice. Also, having practised the *Establishing the Meditation Frame* technique sufficiently, there will be an appropriate level of robustness, comfort and familiarity with meditation. However, for this reason, the importance of learning meditation with others and under instruction from someone experienced is invaluable as offering another source of support, similar to a supervisor with clinical therapeutic work.

The process of meditation gives the mind a position from which it can develop a closer analysis of different mental states and cut through the background flow of thoughts, feelings, sensations and perceptions. The mind is at a more receptive and refined place with fewer thoughts and fantasies. The ones that do arise are more pertinent to the current situation and the mind is more attuned to the presenting object. In the consultation room, this enables the therapist to be more receptive to the client's unconsciousness with an increased awareness of the therapist's own countertransference.

When thoughts and feelings do arise, the mind does not get caught up in them as readily. Much like a car passing when going for a walk, one can notice it and its characteristics without having to get in and be driven away. In a similar way, one can develop this mode of attention without thoughts running away with themselves. Unlike the type of attention required for evenly suspended attention, this is a more open rather than focussed level of concentration. The mind must be receptive to a range of experiences. It is the role of the therapist's own analysis to develop the ability to distinguish whether these arising issues are their own or coming from the client. However, meditation can help to increase sensitivity and build an internal stance that can support recognition with consequential analysis instead of unconscious action. An important feature is to ensure that in an attempt to maintain a meditation, concentration does not become too focussed which would risk blocking out these experiences.

> Since, however, violent emotions of any kind, of love or hate, helpfulness or anger, impel towards action rather than towards contemplation and blur a person's capacity to observe and weigh the evidence correctly, it follows that, if the analyst's emotional response is intense, it will defeat its object.
>
> Therefore the analyst's emotional sensitivity needs to be extensive rather than intensive, differentiating and mobile.
>
> (Heimann, 1950, p. 82)

Meditation helps to create this internal setting allowing the mind to be far-ranging without getting bogged down in the emotional weight of the countertransference. The technique depicted below supports the therapist to experience, yet remain at a sufficient distance from, their countertransferential experience.

It can also be helpful to have a way of understanding and categorising the countertransference. This can be firstly noticed by virtue of the mode of the experience. So, for example is it a thought, sensation, feeling or fantasy. Racker gave a few more categories specific to the relationship of the countertransference with the client. The first, concordant identification points to if the countertransference is identified with the client's id or ego and the therapist is experiencing the same thing as the client – they are experiencing the same inner reality. This concordant countertransference is the core of how empathy emerges and is based on projection and identification. In contrast, while complementary countertransference is also based on projection and identification, the client treats the therapist as an internal object and the therapist feels as if they are being projected into as if an earlier or other relationship is being replayed between them (Racker, 1957).

The same opening technique is utilised in establishing the meditation frame, followed by the method in the development of evenly suspended attention. After evenly suspended attention has been established, which could take a fair amount of time depending on the experience of the meditator, we will expand the awareness beyond the breath. Instead of staying at that point and returning to the breath when the mind wanders to different thoughts, sensations and feelings, these are the very grist for the mill of this technique.

The measure of readiness to move on from the evenly suspended stage can be gauged by whether the mind is focussed enough to be able to sustain the second stage of this technique. Therefore, it is an iterative process whereby it might be necessary to return to the evenly suspended attention around the breath if the mind becomes too easily lost in these experiences that are occurring beyond the breath. After having practised for sufficient time, you will develop the necessary awareness to know when to move on from this stage of the practice without having to go back and forth, and it might also move much faster depending on your state of mind. Experiment with yourself, and you can change your technique accordingly. Bear in mind, too, that on a given day or time, it may simply not be possible to reach certain points in your practice. Without getting too frustrated, accept the situation and move to a practice which is more comfortable and possible. Meditation practice and its fruits are developed over a long period of time. Consistency and frequency are more important than single sessions, being able to sit for a single long period of time or practising in a particular way.

When a thought or feeling comes into the mind, rather than using mindfulness to return to the breath immediately, a mental note should be made and its nature explored. This technique forms the basis of developing an increased alertness to thoughts, feelings, perceptions and sensations as they arise. Indeed, the awareness of the body and the arising thoughts and feelings go hand in hand. As discussed in the introduction, the breath being on the cusp between the conscious and unconscious is also affected by the thoughts and feelings that we experience. Therefore, increased alertness to one goes hand in hand with the other. This concept of noting and investigation brings in other aspects of conscious analysis to the process of meditation and once again, steers us away from one of the preconceptions around meditation that the aim is a state where no thoughts occur. Instead, we can see how our awareness can occupy different parts of the mind – move with it at times and at other times ana-lyse what happened. A bit like a boat in the sea, we can drift with the tide if the direction is favourable before using the sail, engine and rudder to make our own way as necessary.

Having developed the technique outlined at the end of the chapter, it should become easier to notice changes within the body when certain feelings arise, such as the tensions held when anger arises – tension in the neck or the jaw, or the bodily experience of empathy –warmth in the chest, fullness behind the eyes or pressure at the throat. These experiences will always express themselves on the breath and throughout the body but often go unnoticed. Therefore, a greater sensitivity and alertness towards how the mind and body are affected by an object can be cultivated and consequentially, an increased awareness of countertransferential experiences as they arise in the consultation room or later when thinking about the client and session that has occurred. While the meditation exercise described here is more of a passive one – seeing what arises, we will also explore how a more active body scanning meditation can support us to discover how we might have particular physical countertransferential responses in the chapter on *Body-Centred Psychotherapy – Somatic Perspectives*.

After this first stage of recognising the arising experiences, we will use evaluating awareness to consider and discern whether they are arising from the meditation itself or externally. For example, the in-breath causing an experience of relaxation, or perhaps increased anxiety from physical pain due to being uncomfortable in comparison to whether the experience is from another source, perhaps a desire or concern from outside the meditation. The ability to discern whether these experiences come from the object or elsewhere can also support the faculty of differentiating a countertransferential experience as concordant or complementary. We could point towards that experience relating to the meditation, so with the object itself, as concordant – a sort of empathy with another part of ourselves or complementary – an external or past relationship being brought in. Once this evaluation has been completed under the spotlight of sufficiently focussed concentration, the practice can return to the first stage of this technique, awaiting for arising experiences, noticing and then evaluating them. If an overwhelming amount of experiences arise, then it is best to stay with the first stage to develop further focus.

Therefore, from first stage of the technique to the second we move towards more open awareness, in order to open up to different experiences. In a similar way, the technique moves from the non-judgemental evenly suspended state to an increasingly evaluating awareness of the discernment range. In the first stage, the factor of alertness and mindfulness takes the most active part and in the second stage alertness is more predominate assuming the mind is focussed enough as it's focussing on the here and now. Throughout the technique ardency is used to develop the mental qualities required to be able to be focussed and evaluate what is happening as well as adjusting and changing when this may not be happening.

This meditation technique helps to develop the faculty of tolerating the intense feelings that arise in the consultation room, observe them without acting on and use them as material to understand the mind. Strong feelings and sensations arise in meditation and it is up to the meditator to recognise and evaluate them abstaining from acting out. By extension, this internal setting can be used in the consulting room where the client's unconscious becomes the object. From a well-developed meditation practice there is the ability to tolerate a client's projective identifications, distress and when encountering clients with more aggressive ways of communicating. Perhaps a thought or feeling about the material that arises may fill the mind with an urgency to take action. Meditation can help with the ability to use the mind's own resources to stick with the frame and stay until the end of the allotted time without acting on these feelings. When unusual things happen in a session, there can be the necessary space in the mind to think about what occurred with a client rather than immediately respond to the event. Instead, we can metabolise them and make a meaningful interpretation or contain the client's experience without potentially repeating ways in which a client usually relates and draws out responses from others. This can bolster that initial general therapeutic stance as a container, maintaining boundaries and creating a holding environment as described earlier in the book.

Meditation Exercise – Developing Internal Listening, Countertransference

This meditation exercise follows from *Establishing the Meditation Frame* and *Developing External Listening, Evenly Suspended Attention*.

After having established the meditation frame and an evenly suspended attention, we will turn our awareness to a more open stance in order to observe, note and analyse sequentially the different experiences that may arise. We take our attention from the breath, open and expand awareness to observe across all sensory modalities, thoughts, feelings and fantasies, turning our attention to whatever may arise. Once something does arise, we will make a mental note of what it might be. This is as simple as using the inner voice to say *thinking*, *gladness* or *feeling pains*. After noting, we move to analyse – noticing and naming where this experience might be coming from. This can be the most challenging part, but we will try to keep it brief assessing whether it comes from the meditation experience itself – a parallel to concordant countertransference or an issue exterior to the meditation – an equivalent of concurrent countertransference. We can take things one more step beyond that with a theory of what might be underlying this experience, for example, stress to do with work demands. The aim, however, is not one of self-therapy but limited to this sequential process of observing, noting and analysis. The mind will inevitably get side-tracked and too absorbed by one of these experiences. The aim is to try to become aware, notice and observe what is happening at as early an opportunity as possible in order to note and analyse it. If the mind or body is feeling too chaotic and unsettled then it might be necessary to return to one of the earlier stages of meditation or use the breath to focus the mind.

Expand Awareness → Notice → Note → Analyse Nature → Suggest Source

When you have completed the meditation, open your eyes and spend a few minutes reviewing the session. Some questions on which to reflect:

◆ What was it like shifting between the different aspects of the meditation?
◆ How are you left feeling at the end of the meditation, maybe less calm than other meditations having had some experiences stirred up?
◆ Did you find yourself returning to the breath often?
◆ If this wasn't the first time trying this, did you stay with the latter parts of the exercise more than before?

Reveries

Sit in reverie and watch the changing colour of the waves that break upon the idle seashore of the mind.

(Longfellow, 1844, p. 50)

As described early in the book, Bion introduced the idea of the therapist's reverie as equivalent to the state of mind of the mother who can make sense and contain the raw experiences of the infant who cannot process them with their own mind. More recent work, which we will explore, has expanded this idea into something akin to a "dreamlike flash" (Ferro and Basile, 2004). and "the waking dream thought" denoting them as reveries (Ferro, 2006). We will explore how we can engender a similar mindset analogous to a kind of daydreaming or volitional mind-wandering that can make the therapist more aware and receptive to these reveries.

I am also conscious of the work of Thomas Ogden regarding reveries, who describes them as "a motley collection of psychological states that seem to reflect the analyst's narcissistic self-absorption ... daydreaming" (Ogden, 2004). However, in agreement with Birksted-Breen (2016) who describes this closer to Winnicott's "fantasying," I would suggest they would fit closer with the previous chapter on countertransferential experiences, or even as the free associations of the therapist albeit with a wider frame of reference. Indeed, Ogden groups countertransference reactions as reveries. For this reason, in this section, I'll be looking at the post-Bion psychoanalysts – Ferro (an Italian psychoanalyst) and the da Rocha Barroses (Elizabeth L. and Elias M. – Brazilian psychoanalysts) as well as using the excellent summaries from Fred Busch (an American psychoanalyst) on this potentially challenging concept. I find their more specific definitions and explorations of reveries are more clearly distinguished from the previous chapter on countertransference.

Ferro postulates that a dream-like image comes into the mind of the therapist as a communication from the client in the form of a pictogram which has an associated affect. This represents the undigested experience of the client communicated to the therapist through a projective identification. Ferro finds that the experiencing of the pictographic impression and the development of this capacity is in itself fulfilling the process for the metabolising of the more primitive states that the client has expressed – that of a container. Ferro understands the pictographic process to be a continuous activity which itself is the mind's way of processing all stimuli and it is:

> ... the centrality of the metabolizing activity we carry out on any and all sensorial and psychological impressions (occurs via) ... forming a visual pictograph or ideogram from every stimulus, in other words a poetic image that synchronizes the emotional result of each stimulus or set of stimuli.
>
> (Ferro, 2002)

The pictogram is a surprising, flash of an image that has a dream-like quality. I think of it as that spark of inspiration that might occur after being puzzled by something or a moment of clarity loaded with emotional content all conjured up into an image in the mind's eye. Unlike more narrative-based free associations, reveries have a more dream-like quality by virtue of this pictographic and sense impression nature. For the Da Rocha Barroses, it is the symbolising of these reveries to the client which completes the cycle of reverie as described by Bion and in my opinion is closer to that description. In comparison, I find it harder with Ferro's understanding, to bridge the gap between the therapist's experience and how the client then receives back the communication other than through some kind of general unconscious process of introjection. Also, with Ferro's concept of reveries, more of the weight of psychic processing for the client lands on the therapist's shoulders. My experience has been more that there is a collaborative experience with more of an exchange, although depending on the client's functioning and ability to process their own distress, this varies from person to person.

Due to this, I prefer the approach the Da Rocha Barroses make when they describe that by processing and then symbolising the experience, the therapist makes it more explicit as a translation into a symbol as an interpretation rather than a more general interpretative activity that rests more with the therapist. Busch emphasises this symbol to be expressed as an actual interpretation to clients which offers us what feels to be a more practical application, especially when thinking about how meditation method might be derived as an expression of this process (Busch, 2019).

The Da Rocha Barroses stress:

> ... the idea that the process itself of constructing the symbol in its different components and its vicissitudes is centrally important to contemporary psychoanalysis since symbols are essential for thinking and for storing emotional experiences in our memory and for conveying our affects to others and make them explicit for ourselves.
> (Da Rocha Barros and Da Rocha Barros, 2011, p.879)

They then describe the importance of analysing and then interpreting the reverie back to the client:

> Before building his interpretation it is necessary for the analyst to go through a complex psychic working through, in part conscious, in part not. It is not enough for him to be aware of what feelings are projected into his mind by the patient; he also needs to trace back in what way the experience of these feelings have affected him. This second stage is essential to make efficient usage of reverie and to characterize it conceptually as such. The identification of this experience, in self-analysis, allows the analyst to apprehend the aspect of the patient that is dynamically unavailable. This process bears a certain similarity to what happens in dream production. We think the expression "to dream the patient's dream" (Cassorla, 2013) is born out from this situation.
> (Da Rocha Barros and Da Rocha Barros, 2016, p. 148)

The next step entails an effort by the analyst to put into words (that is, in discursive symbolic form) that which will be communicated as an interpretation/observation (response to the longing for language, the search for the sayable) addressed to the patient. These are not just casual words, but those aspiring to produce an emotional experience of insight (that creates new links), which generate in the patient a live feeling of "Ah, this makes sense and allows me to understand the meaning of this instance in my life and associate it with other moments."

(Da Rocha Barros and Da Rocha Barros, 2016, p. 149)

So, how to contrast these reveries with the experience of countertransference as described above? It is the dream-like state that the therapist embodies combined with the sudden or flash like appearance of the image into the mind imbued with a strong emotional content. There is a less formal analysis of this experience and more of a sort of *bubbling up* representing the metabolising of the client's projective identification. Therefore, it emerges from a position *without memory or desire* as opposed to one closer to evenly suspended attention. It is less the therapist as a mirror that Freud described as reflecting the client's experience and closer to an involvement with the client. In his comparative study of different post-Bionian positions on reveries, Busch emphasises the importance of a self-reflective process following the emergence of a reverie:

The post-Bionians are brilliant in seeing what comes to mind, but those like Ogden seem not to reflect on why what comes to mind comes to mind, as he sees himself in a state of reverie where everything he thinks is a reverie. Self-reflection, with all of its problems as a source of information about what is on our mind, is the analyst's one bullwork against self-deception.

(Busch, 2018)

Thus, we arrive at a similar process to that of experiencing countertransference, but with a different mindset and quality of experience, something more ineffable and dreamlike, which perhaps while might be harder to grasp in words I hope my clinical example below will illustrate.

We can then move to think about how reveries can be experienced through a meditation embodying that dream-like position. This can take the form of volitional mind wandering which has been shown to be supportive of making meaning of the world and increasing an understanding of relationships. This sort of mind wandering creates a decoupling from external tasks and perceptions and it has been suggested can offer a more satisfying internal mental life with increased creativity, problem solving and enhanced social skills (McMillan, Kaufman and Singer, 2013). While we might be very familiar with this position of mind wandering or decoupling akin to daydreaming, I would not say it is meditation itself because of the absence of mindfulness and alertness. However, if coupled with some mindfulness to bring attention back after a process of volitional mind wandering and consequential reverie, we could see how a state of mind that is fertile for the emergence of reveries may be developed. If this process is also employed when having a specific client or piece of clinical experience in mind, then it can be seen how the reveries may be more closely related to that client.

The technique will, therefore, have three stages – first, visualising a specific client, a session with a client or even specific interaction within one session so that any emerging reveries have an association with clinical work. We will then allow the mind to wander off and either let the process take its course or use an alarm after a couple of minutes, we will then mindfully bring our attention back and, being alert, notice what has emerged. For there to be a difference between the previously described countertransferential experience then the mind wandering element has to truly enter into a more unfocussed, open and dreamlike mode.

Reveries and Breathwork in the Consultation Room

The following clinical example has been appropriately anonymised to prevent the identification of the patient while preserving the crux of the interaction. I hope it illustrates both the emergence as use of a reverie with a client and also how a meditation technique used in the session can support this. This type of *in session* breathwork will be explored more in the *Other Complementary Techniques* chapter.

Mrs A is in her 50s. She presented for once-a-week psychodynamic psychotherapy with long-standing depression characterised by intense self-loathing and suicidal ideation. Mrs A appeared to be high functioning and working in a supportive non-clinical role for a local hospital. She previously had worked as a police officer. Mrs A used cannabis to manage her mood and stress, albeit under the guise of regulating her sleep. Mrs A had online sexual relationships with men behind her husband's back, which she justified as preventing her from leaving him.

Mrs A's initial presentation in the consulting room was characterised by narcissism and she would attack me and the therapy. During the first months, Mrs A would stare into my eyes at length, which she consequentially denied. In a time of more insight, Mrs A had described that this was a test which she regretted, thinking it was childish and feeling some guilt. However, this was temporary and as we got more in touch with feelings of guilt around her erratic behaviour associated with cannabis use, or her online relationships, she would become more attacking. It was very difficult for Mrs A to get in touch with envy which was a key aspect to her difficulties and would strongly deny any transference interpretations saying that they must be because of issues I have. Mrs A would make demands from me to ask more direct questions and give the therapy more direction. She became frustrated that she could not *figure things out* without help, often coming back to the phrase *the cobbler's children have no shoes* that she, as someone who works in a hospital environment, should be able to treat and cure herself without assistance.

In one particular session, Mrs A was left feeling very angry, accusing me of not *giving a straight answer to a straight question* when I had interpreted rather than answered direct questions about what practical actions she should take to bring about change in her life. Mrs A returned to the thought that she wanted therapy to *walk the walk not just talk the talk* diminishing our work to a conversation with no meaningful outcome. She then returned to stare directly into my eyes.

It was challenging to maintain an evenly suspended stance at this point due to the power of the projections coming from Mrs A, who was seemingly calm and collected but had effectively emptied out her anger and feelings of despair at being exposed to her anxieties into me. It felt potentially overwhelming, so I consciously took a breath so I could engage myself in a state of negative capability and also maintain my therapeutic stance. This brought about an increase in focus and non-judgemental awareness. Another breath enabled me to open my concentration to allow in the feelings and experiences that had previously felt like one overwhelming block. My discernment shifted to an evaluating one to be able to think about the feelings and what they might mean rather than unconsciously act on them.

I will now describe the affective journey that I went on. I felt very lonely and angry as if I were the only person in the room thinking about what was happening. The anger had an indignant element and also a sense of being forced down a one-way street without a choice. It was as if it were my fault Mrs A felt like this and the only way out was for me to satisfy her various demands to alleviate her anxiety. It was at this point that an image quickly arrived into my mind's eye of a one-lane highway with a car being driven at great speed ahead of me, my visual field being dragged ahead in its wake. The phrase *my way or the highway* came into my mind as an expression of this pictogram. With the arrival of this image and the phrase came a change in my affect, a sort of cooling as if the anger and frustration had dissipated somewhat.

I put it to Mrs A that this was how she could sometimes interact with others, such as she had with myself incorporating the phrase *my way or the highway* into my interpretation. This really resonated with Mrs A and became somewhat of a *leitmotif* which seemingly replaced some of the aforementioned phrases to which Mrs A would often return. Mrs A's affect and body language shifted. She became pensive, looking away, and repeated the phrase back to me and herself a few times. She proceeded to get in touch with her guilt and concern about how her behaviour had affected her family through her cannabis use and online sexual interactions with men.

I think this interpretation cut through, as it spoke to Bion's initial description of reverie as "the state of mind which is open to the reception of any "object" from the loved object and is therefore capable of the reception of the infant's projective identifications whether they are felt to be good or bad" (Bion, 1962, p. 36) with the consequential transformation of those projections into something palatable for the infant or patient to then reintroject.

By tolerating the attack and helping Mrs A make sense of it in this way, I offered a new way of relating without either Mrs A being the subject of attack from another, or experiencing persecutory guilt about her initial attack. The experience of the reverie – which had this dream-like quality imbued with the range of emotions I described, combined with a symbolisation and interpretation as described above by the Da Rocha Barroses gave an intersubjective processing of Mrs. A's experience and crucially an understanding and meaning for her. Without the conscious breaths imbued with meaning from meditation, I think it would have been harder to tolerate this situation, be open to experiencing the reverie and arrive at such a meaningful interpretation in the moment.

Meditation Exercise – Developing Internal Listening, Reveries

Before beginning the meditation, try to think of a specific client, recent session or interaction with a client. Next, progress through the meditation exercises *Establishing the Meditation Frame* and *Developing External Listening, Without Memory or Desire and Negative Capability*. The focus of this meditation will be to get into a state of mind where reveries arise and notice the process occurring. If you would like, set an alarm to ring every five minutes if you think that it will be too challenging to be able to catch yourself when your mind has been wandering. Bring into your mind's eye the particular person or scenario that you have thought of earlier. Take some time to picture this, focussing on the boundaries of the situation – the physical situation including the room and where you are both positioned, what they look like, what it feels like to be with them, what words were said between you both and your emotional experience there. If the words being said form a short sentence or series of exchanges, try repeating them within your mind a few times. After staying with this experience, try to allow your mind to decouple from it, let your alertness drop off and the mind to wander off on its own course into the reveries.

Then, either after the alarm goes off, or when the mind emerges from this reverie take a mental note of what happened, of what scenario came into your mind, image, phrase, sensation or emotion. Give yourself three sighs to establish your alertness on the breaths and your current state of mind and ardency to sit in reverie and drop your focus. See if you can aim to immerse yourself even more fully in the experience of your reveries and, although maybe counterintuitive, abandon your mindfulness for a period of time. While your mind goes into this state, see if you can still have one part observing what is going on, if you completely lose your awareness, then it can be hard both to emerge from it and also remember where your mind actually went. Therefore, there is still some alertness still present throughout. It can be hard to keep this balance. You will know if you have reached it when you manage to return your awareness fully and still recollect most of the reverie.

When you have completed a few rounds of this, take a moment to bring yourself back to the room. It can be helpful to make a note of the reveries that emerged as associated with the clinical material that was visualised. You can then use this to be reviewed in supervision or reflected upon. This exercise can also be practised just before a session with a client to create a more fertile environment for reveries to emerge with the client at the time. This can be the most challenging aspect of the clinical application of reveries and also using countertransferential experiences in the room with a client. If they are more accessible to conscious awareness generally, then it gives us more of a chance to be able to use the experiences with clients in a contemporaneous way and for this reason a meditation exercise such as this can be supportive.

- ◆ Did you find you were able to shift your mindset between the different positions effectively?
- ◆ Did you find yourself getting a bit too lost in the reveries or could you bring yourself back OK?
- ◆ Can you make a connection between the initial piece of clinical material, your volitional mind wandering and reveries?

Chapter Summary

- ◆ Getting in touch with countertransference and working with reveries form the mindsets that make up the internal listening approaches involved in the psychoanalytic stance
- ◆ Greater sensitivity to countertransference can be developed using a noting meditation method
- ◆ Getting access to reveries can be enhanced through a process of volitional mind wandering followed by mindfully returning to a state of alertness and later analysis
- ◆ A clinical example is brought in to illustrate the sometimes elusive concept of reveries as well as give a taste of how breathwork can be brought into the consultation room.

References

Bion, W.R. (1959). Attacks on linking. *The International Journal of Psychoanalysis*, 40, pp.308–315.

Bion, W.R. (1962). *Learning from Experience*. London: Heinemann.

Birksted-Breen, D. (2016). Bi-ocularity, the functioning mind of the psychoanalyst. *The International Journal of Psychoanalysis*, 97(1), pp.25–40.

Brenman Pick, I. (1985). Working through in the countertransference. *The International Journal of Psychoanalysis*, 66, pp.157–166.

Busch, F. (2018). Searching for the analyst's reveries. *The International Journal of Psychoanalysis*, 99(3), pp.569–589.

Busch, F. (2019). *The Analyst's Reveries Explorations in Bion's Enigmatic Concept*. Oxford: Routledge.

Carpy, D.V. (1989). Tolerating the countertransference: A mutative process. *The International Journal of Psychoanalysis*, 70, pp.287–294.

Cassorla, R. (2013). In search of symbolization: The analyst's task of dreaming. In: *Unrepresented States and the Construction of Meaning*. London: Karnac.

Da Rocha Barros, E.M. and Da Rocha Barros, E.L. (2011). Reflections on the clinical implications of symbolism. *The International Journal of Psychoanalysis*, 92(4), pp.879–901.

Da Rocha Barros, E.M. and Da Rocha Barros, E.L. (2016). The function of evocation in the working- through of the countertransference: Projective identification, reverie, and the expressive function of the mind-reflections inspired by Bion's work. In H. Levine and G. Civitarese (Eds.), *The Bion Tradition* (141–154). London: Karnac.

Ferro, A. (2002). Narrative derivatives of alpha elements: Clinical implications. *International Forum of Psychoanalysis*, 11(3), pp.184–187.

Ferro, A. (2006). Trauma, reverie, and the field. *Psychoanalytic Quarterly*, 75(4), pp.1045–1056.

Ferro, A. and Basile, R. (2004). The psychoanalyst as individual: Self-analysis and gradients of functioning. *The Psychoanalytic Quarterly*, 73(3), pp.659–682.

Gallese, V. (2009). Mirror neurons, embodied simulation, and the neural basis of social identification. *Psychoanalytic Dialogues*, 19(5), pp.519–536.

Gallese, V., Eagle, M.N. and Migone, P. (2007). Intentional attunement: Mirror neurons and the neural underpinnings of interpersonal relations. *Journal of the American Psychoanalytic Association*, 55(1), pp.131–175.

Heimann, P. (1950). On countertransference. *The International Journal of Psychoanalysis*, 31, pp.81–84.

Hickok, G. (2009). Eight problems for the mirror neuron theory of action understanding in monkeys and humans. *Journal of Cognitive Neuroscience*, 21(7), pp.1229–1243.

Iacoboni, M. (2009). Imitation, empathy, and mirror neurons. *Annual Review of Psychology*, 60(1), pp.653–670.

Klein, M. (1946). Notes on some schizoid mechanisms. *The International Journal of Psychoanalysis*, 27, pp.99–110.

Longfellow, H.W. (1844). *The Spanish Student: A Play in Three Acts*. Cambridge: John Owen.

McMillan, R.L., Kaufman, S.B. and Singer, J.L. (2013). Ode to positive constructive daydreaming. *Frontiers in Psychology*, 4.

Ogden, T.H. (2004). The analytic third: Implications for psychoanalytic theory and technique. *The Psychoanalytic Quarterly*, 73(1), pp.167–195.

Parsons, M. (2007). Raiding the inarticulate: The internal analytic setting and listening beyond countertransference. *The International Journal of Psychoanalysis*, 88(6), pp.1441–1456.

Piedfort-Marin, O. (2018). Transference and countertransference in EMDR therapy. *Journal of EMDR Practice and Research*, 12(3), pp.158–172.

Pizzamiglio, L., Aprile, T., Spitoni, G., Pitzalis, S., Bates, E., D'Amico, S. and Di Russo, F. (2005). Separate neural systems for processing action- or non-action-related sounds. *NeuroImage*, 24(3), pp.852–861.

Popper, K. (1963). *Conjectures and Refutations: The Growth of Scientific Knowledge*. London: Routledge.

Racker, H. (1957). The meanings and uses of countertransference. *The Psychoanalytic Quarterly*, 26(3), pp.303–357.

Rizzolatti, G., Fadiga, L., Gallese, V. and Fogassi, L. (1996). Premotor cortex and the recognition of motor actions. *Cognitive Brain Research*, 3(2), pp.131–141.

Schermer, V.L. (2010). Mirror neurons: Their implications for group psychotherapy. *International Journal of Group Psychotherapy*, 60(4), pp.486–513.

Vivona, J.M. (2009). Leaping from brain to mind: A critique of mirror neuron explanations of countertransference. *Journal of the American Psychoanalytic Association*, 57(3), pp.525–550.

5 Body-Centred Psychotherapy

Somatic Perspectives

Body-Centred Countertransference

The body-centred psychotherapies, also known as somatic or simply body psychotherapies, encompass a range of therapies which are all defined by their focus on the body of the client and also as we will be exploring in this chapter that of the therapist too. Starting as many modalities do from work by Sigmund Freud, Wilhelm Reich (1897–1957) an Austrian medical doctor and psychoanalyst is most often thought of as bringing this focus on the body into his work more explicitly, alongside Fritz Perls (1893–1970) a German psychiatrist and psychoanalyst with his development of Gestalt therapy. Historically, as with many of the earlier developments in psychotherapy, body psycho-therapy was rejected by more mainstream psychoanalytic and behavioural approaches. In contemporary therapeutic practice techniques involving a focus on the body are practised widely and often integratively alongside other approaches. Interest in the connections between mind and body in trauma has more recently found a place in more popular psychological thinking due to the work of Bessel van der Kolk (2014). Nowadays, there is a wide range of psychotherapy modalities all loosely associated through this grounding in Reichian thought and practice which Totton (2003) sorts into the categories of Reichian, primal, trauma,

DOI: 10.4324/9781003382959-5

process, expressive and integrative therapies, each with their own emphases on theory and praxis.

In this chapter, we will focus on why and how the experience of the therapist's body can be so important in working with clients in a more body-focussed way. In body-centred psychotherapies, countertransference is particularly felt through the therapist's bodily experience such is the nature of this kind of therapy, where the body takes on a more prominent significance. That's not to say that the body is not relevant in many if not all of the therapy modalities that are discussed in this book, but that cognitive and affective domains often dominate in the way that clients are understood and the techniques that a therapist might use. There is also evidence that the essential nature of meditation is one with a somatic core primarily concerned with the regulation of the mind when it wanders from a focus on the body. This in turn leads to enhanced cognitive processes as a product of organising the flow of sensory information in the brain (Kerr et al., 2013). So, as with the somatic psychotherapies, the body can be viewed as of primary importance in meditation.

There is a vast range in the way that people might experience a bodily sensation in response to an emotional stimulus. The connection between 100 core feelings from 1026 participants has been mapped onto images of bodies using both bodily sensation mapping and a neuroimaging meta-analysis (Nummenmaa et al., 2018). This produces a fascinating visual representation of how people experience feelings within their own bodies. So, for example, tiredness is mainly felt in the head, guilt has hotspots in the head and chest area, fear through the head and torso and relaxation is much more diffused throughout the body. Therefore, while one can draw conclusions about how an average person may physically experience a feeling or thought, nearly all of the maps show some level of distribution into other areas of the body. This shows there is a spectrum of individual experience informed not only by personal histories but also by various cultural influences depending on more geographically localised somatic experiences combined with cognitive of affective phenomena. For example, in France, the experience of heavy legs as a somatic experience of physical or emotional stress is common, yet cross over the English Channel to the United Kingdom and this is almost unheard of.

Bringing things more specifically to the experience of psychotherapists, a study of 84 psychologists and their experiences of body-centred countertransference (those somatic phenomena which a therapist experiences associated with the presence of a client) found a range of experiences (listed in decreasing frequency) including sleepiness, muscle tension, unexpected shift in body, yawning, tearfulness, headaches, stomach disturbance, aches in joints, throat constriction, loss of voice, raised voice, numbness, dizziness, sexual arousal, nausea and genital pain. This shows the real range of experiences that can occur for therapists. After taking into account a host of confounding factors, the researchers found it was how the psychologists engaged with the countertransference and responded to it which determined the effects on the therapy. They emphasised the importance of normalising and discussing these experiences to reduce the risks of acting on these particularly powerful phenomena (Egan and Carr, 2008).

The importance of somatic countertransference in body-centred psychotherapy and beyond is summed up as follows:

> Whether we call it 'somatic' or 'embodied' counter-transference, 'somatic resonance', 'somatic empathy', 'dreaming up', or something else, this capacity for embodied relationship – including all of the irrational and projective elements of relationship in general – is a tremendously important tool for body psychotherapy …
> It can be argued that the use of somatic countertransference, with no other specifically body-oriented tools, is in itself sufficient to qualify the work as body psychotherapy (Roz Carroll, personal communication).
>
> (Totton, 2003, p. 87)

Clinically, as with other forms of countertransference, it has a particularly powerful way of cutting through in terms of providing information beyond those more apparent verbal communications from a client. As experienced through the body, it can offer a more immediate understanding, requiring fewer layers of self-interpretation to understand the communication compared to cognitive or affective forms of countertransference. This is illustrated with a description of concordant somatic countertransference:

> I very often get 'symptoms' when a patient begins a session or after some moments of work. These are usually bodily reactions of various kinds, such as headaches, stomach aches, heartaches, shortness of breath, sphincter tensions, fatigue, etc. They do not usually have a direct connection with what is being said, but whenever I reveal these reactions, I almost always discover that the patient is having, or had in the recent past, the same symptom or one related to it. Most of the time an underlying symbolic parallel is associated to the psychological content being discussed.
>
> (Spiegelman, 1996, p. 114 in Totton, 2003, p. 85)

The importance of the awareness of somatic countertransference experiences can help in the process of mirroring a client in body psychotherapy, a technique which supports the client in their emotional processing:

> Somatic countertransference is particularly complicated when therapists join with, or "match," their clients, unconsciously imitating their physical posture and movements. If mirroring is done without mindful awareness, the therapist may "take on" the client's tension, arousal, movement, and posture without realizing it, which in turn affects the cognitive and emotional levels of processing. On the other hand, deliberate mirroring can provide the therapist with valuable information about the client's physical tendencies and help the client feel empathic rapport with the therapist.
>
> (Ogden, Minton and Pain, 2006, p. 174)

Therefore, it is important to tread carefully and be conscious of the body, not just what is being said, but how the body of the therapist may be communicating to the client a variety of messages. Awareness of these subtle interactions can prevent the unintentional consequences of unconsciously responding to a client through the body:

> If countertransference and their somatic tendencies go unrecognized, therapists are at risk of acting on these tendencies. It is the therapist's responsibility to address his or her countertransference through self-awareness and supervision, so that it can function as an asset rather than a liability in therapy. Transference responses are also expected and desired; the particular physical and mental action tendencies that accompany them provide an opportunity for both greater awareness about these dynamics and a corrective emotional and developmental experience for the client.
>
> (Ogden, Minton and Pain, 2006, p. 175)

Therefore, in addition to gaining more clinical experience, learning through supervision and one's own therapy, meditation offers another avenue by which a therapist may be able to get more in touch with their own bodies. What is known as a *body scanning* meditation technique can be used to increase sensitivity and also become more conscious of what bodily experiences may be particular to a given therapist. It can then be possible to engage more sensitively and meaningfully with the body, offering greater access to a crucial tool in understanding clients and their communications on a somatic level. This meditation method also allows us to become more accustomed to the various physical processes that are constantly occurring but are outside of our immediate awareness on a more preconscious level. Therefore, when more gross somatic experiences arise through the process of working with a client, they might feel less alarming making it more possible to think rather than react.

The body scanning meditation technique outlined below is used to direct awareness in a systematic way throughout the whole of the body from head to toe. Initially, this is performed with awareness focussing on the skin and what feelings may arise in various locations. The different areas being focussed on start with a larger section, for example, detecting any sensation on the entire head. Then, the focus is progressively reduced to smaller and smaller parts, such as the front of the face, to the nose, and then just the tip of the nose. Once sensitivity and focus increase, the awareness can move or flow across the skin like a wave or as the name suggests a scan. We can then also become sensitive to internal bodily experiences. As the list above suggests, much of the somatic countertransference is felt viscerally, within the body, such as the stomach or joints. Awareness of these parts of the body is joined together into a full scan of the external and internal of the skin and more visceral sensations.

Countertransference has been explored earlier in the book with a meditation method which relies on increasing sensitivity when it is located predominately in the mind. A meditation technique such as body scanning can bring a more active searching faculty whereby an internal listening to bodily experiences serves as a reflection of a mental state. Therefore, it isn't just creating sensitivity but also an increased capacity to find these bodily experiences. I came to a body-scanning technique after much time meditating with methods which are seemingly less active – more open, non-judgemental awareness practices where the experience unfolds in front of you without interference, but also without directing attention towards anything in particular. It was a breath of fresh air to take on a technique where I felt like I was *doing* more, or more accurately there is an increased role of ardency and effort.

After attending many retreats where the focus of practice is body scanning, I have developed a keener awareness of my body, especially how it reacts to my emotional states and where I might hold stress, anxiety, low mood, compassion, joy or any other number of different feelings. It can be a helpful indicator to me when an affect may not be conscious, and therefore, a powerful tool in terms of countertransference and how it relates to a client. By being more in touch with my body, I am more sensitive to somatic countertransference and also more able to delineate between a concordant or concurrent bodily countertransference experience. Greater awareness of the body also has particular importance for other meditation techniques, especially the *breathing through the body* method, which is the main formal meditation method I regularly practice which I describe closer to the end of the book.

In terms of the meditation framework, the body scan can be seen to utilise mindfulness to remember to remain on the body but driven forward with an ardency that is expressed by the flow of the scan. Alertness is key to noticing and it is this factor which opens up the body to awareness combined with a non-judgemental type of discernment as the sensations arising are not noted to be good or bad, skilful or unskilful, but rather the aim is to increase sensitivity. This type of meditation is particularly effective at developing resilience due to accepting the more challenging feelings of discomfort, such as pains or itches, without ending the meditation early or radically altering posture. Equally, this attitude is turned to the more pleasant experiences that might arise, developing a stance of non-grasping towards them. That said, it is not meant to be a test of grit and if functional pain is present due to an injury or illness, then of course, moving about to be comfortable is more important than staying with an acutely uncomfortable experience.

Concentration is open enough to increase sensitivity to the range of bodily sensations, albeit focussed on this particular modality of bodily sensations at the expense of other domains. If there are expectations about what sensation may be experienced in a specific location or perhaps a hope that a more pleasant flow instead of say pain may be experienced, then it becomes harder to notice what is actually occurring in the body as the mind is pushing its own expectations on reality. For this reason, a high level of focus is also required to carefully move through the different sections of the body. Therefore, in this way, concentration is focussed on the body, but open to the full range of experiences in this particular area.

For some people, it might be too challenging to get in touch with bodily sensations either in all parts of the body or anything beyond the larger, more apparent sensations such as pains or the touch of clothing. For that reason, it can be helpful for these people to try the progressive muscle relaxation technique I have put in the *Other Complementary Techniques* chapter in the first instance. This can sensitise the mind to the more subtle sensations in bodily awareness either by performing it immediately before trying body scanning or as a meditation practice by itself. Another method for people who might find it hard to notice their bodily sensations is to cover the body with more clothing. Many people will meditate underneath a blanket, shawl, or wear an extra hooded sweatshirt. However, once you start to notice, expand and develop your capacity to be aware of your body, the sensitivity will mostly stay.

Meditation Exercise – Developing Somatic Awareness, Body Scanning

After having established the meditation frame, bring your attention to the top of your head. Notice the sensations in your scalp, the touch of the air, and any subtle tingling or pulsing of blood flow which might be more apparent around the temples. Begin to expand your awareness to include the sensations on your forehead, temples, and the space between your eyebrows. Notice any sensation you can before moving on to the next area. When I say any sensation, this can be what I've mentioned, it also includes anything you feel. So, if our attention is on the top of the head or temples it could also be discomfort, pain, itchiness, a dull throb or a sharp pang. Try not just to seek out the more comfortable feelings, or indeed any particular experience else you might not be able to feel anything or could be creating the feelings yourself. Remember that this technique is about discovering whatever sensations might be occurring in the body to open up this realm of experience, instead of just trying to feel something pleasant, which is in effect closing off the range of experience. Therefore, it is an open awareness, albeit focussed within the realm of the body.

Shift your focus to your face. Observe the sensations in your cheeks, nose, lips, and chin. Notice any subtle changes in temperature, tension and any movements within your facial muscles. If possible, focus in on as small an area as possible and move your awareness through your face and onwards like water slowly pouring from the top of your head downwards. While it might at first seem like there is nothing happening, perhaps start with the more apparent feelings associated with the movement of air in and out of the nostrils – the temperature change of cool on inhalation and warmer on exhalation, the flaring of the nostrils with each breath and the sensations of the movement of air on the upper lip. After this, you may feel more sensitised to the other areas of the face. If it is only possible to feel something in one part of the face or one section of the whole head, then accept this is the level of sensitivity at this moment in time and perhaps on the next round, you will notice a sensation appearing in more locations.

Now, direct your attention to your neck and throat. Feel the sensations on the surface of your skin and the deeper sensations within your throat, the inside of your oesophagus (gullet) and the trachea (windpipe), where you would feel food being swallowed and air moving. Notice the subtle movements and sensations as you swallow saliva in the throat and the movement of air as you breathe. Move your attention in a downward direction, either first with your attention on your skin and then inside the body or both at the same time.

If there are any areas of discomfort or tension, see if you can map out the edges of it and notice any inconsistencies in the sensations around or within it. Track where the epicentre seems to be, if it's a constant or pulsing sensation. Notice if your awareness alters the experience of that area – does it become more uncomfortable or dissipate? Does your awareness increase the size of the area, or do you find its edges become more ill-defined?

Bring your awareness to your shoulders. Notice any sensations in this area, the feeling of any clothing on the skin, temperature differences with a perhaps more exposed neck, any tingling or pulsing sensations. Feel the weight of your shoulders as they move – lifting and then dropping away from your ears with each breath.

Now, shift your attention to your arms either one at a time or both at once with your awareness continuing to flow. Feel the sensations on the skin, from the upper arms down to your fingertips. Notice the warmth, coolness, or tingling within your arms. You might find it easier to drill down your focus into smaller and smaller areas. This can be easier to do in the hands where sensitivity is relatively high. Examine each finger from knuckle to tip, both the touch of the fingers where they come into contact with whatever they're resting on, as well as their general feeling. You might notice your blood pulse in your thumbs and fingers if interlaced or at your wrists depending on your hands' position. Again, observe any areas of tension or discomfort, parts that might feel more pleasurable or sections that do not appear to have any sensations.

Direct your focus to your chest and upper back. Notice the sensations on the surface of your skin, the gentle rise and fall of your chest with each breath. Expand your awareness to the deeper sensations within your chest, such as the beating of your heart or the expansion and contraction of your lungs. See if you can notice how these change with each in-breath and out-breath. Again, take some time to map out any areas of tension, discomfort or parts with no sensations, especially around your backbone and the muscles of the back down to the base of the spine.

Now, bring your attention to your abdomen. Notice the sensations in this area as you breathe in and out. Feel the gentle rise and fall of your abdomen with each breath. Observe any subtle movements within your digestive system. Imagine following the path of your food through the digestive system from the stomach through the routes of small and large intestines.

Shift your focus through your lower back, hips and seated area. Notice any sensations or tensions. Feel the contact of your body with the surface beneath you. Bring your awareness to your legs either one by one or both together. Feel the sensations on the skin, from your thighs down to your toes. Notice any areas of warmth, coolness, or tingling. See if you can notice the pulsing of blood flow at contact points with your legs and the floor or chair you are sitting on. Observe the weight of your legs and the contact of your feet with the ground. Allow your legs to feel grounded and relaxed. Follow your attention in this way through each toe on both feet.

Now, turn your attention inward to the interior of your body. Notice the sensations deep within your body, such as what you might think of as a flow of energy, the beating of your heart and blood flow, or the rhythm of your breath. Bring a gentle curiosity to these sensations, allowing them to guide your awareness deeper within.

Now continue either from the tips of the toes back to the top of the head or return to the top of the head and back again. See if, on one round, you can try to notice a sensation in as small an area as possible at each part of the body before moving on to the next small section. If you can't find anything in one spot, try to expand the area until you are able. For example, starting on an area a few centimetres wide and gently expanding. So, if you can't feel the end of the finger, try the whole finger or even the whole hand.

Then, on the next round, see if you can experience something akin to a flow as if a thick liquid is pouring from the top of the body down, or a ring of awareness is encircling the body moving from head to toe. Gradually you will become more familiar with the range of more apparent sensations such as pains, movement, the feeling of clothing or the pressure of limbs on the floor or each other, as well as more subtle sensations that are constantly occurring throughout the body, but are not always within our awareness such as tingling or pulsing as well as the sensations that are occurring within the body too. These can be conceptualised due to the movement of blood, air or food, or in a metaphorical way as a movement of energy within the body.

If it's particularly challenging to be feeling anything in a given area even once you have expanded your attention to, say, the whole limb, then try to gentle tense and then relax one of the muscles in that area. After this, there will surely be a feeling that you can get in touch with. You could then try a smaller area at that section, either with or with the flexing of a muscle. Be patient, it might be some time before a sensation arises, this patience will stand you in good stead and help develop your powers of observation.

- ◆ What was it like mapping out areas that felt more uncomfortable?
- ◆ Did observing them change anything?
- ◆ Did you find you were able to reach an awareness where attention flowed more through the body than just being aware of a part of the body in a more compartmentalised way?
- ◆ How does it feel having finished the meditation, especially in terms of bodily sensations?

Chapter Summary

◆ Body-centred psychotherapies have a particular emphasis on the somatic experience

◆ From the therapist's perspective, an awareness of bodily countertransference is key to both preventing acting in and also bringing insight into the client's experiences

◆ This capacity can be enhanced with the practice of a body scanning meditation technique.

References

Egan, J. and Carr, A. (2008). Body-centred countertransference in female trauma therapists. *Éisteacht*, 8(1), pp.24–27.

Kerr, C.E., Sacchet, M.D., Lazar, S.W., Moore, C.I. and Jones, S.R. (2013). Mindfulness starts with the body: Somatosensory attention and top-down modulation of cortical alpha rhythms in mindfulness meditation. *Frontiers in Human Neuroscience*, 7(12), pp.1–15.

Nummenmaa, L., Hari, R., Hietanen, J.K. and Glerean, E. (2018). Maps of subjective feelings. *Proceedings of the National Academy of Sciences*, 115(37), pp.9198–9203.

Ogden, P., Minton, K. and Pain, C. (2006). *Trauma and the Body: A Sensorimotor Approach to Psychotherapy*. New York, London: W. W. Norton & Company.

Spiegelman, J.M. (1996). *Psychotherapy as Mutual Process*. Scottsdale: New Falcon.

Totton, N. (2003). *Body Psychotherapy An Introduction*. Maidenhead: Open University Press.

van der Kolk, B. (2014). *The Body Keeps the Score: Brain, Mind, and Body in the Healing of Trauma*. New York: Viking Press.

6 Person-Centred Counselling

Unconditional Positive Regard

Unconditional Positive Regard

Carl Rogers (1902–1987), pioneer of humanistic psychology, introduced the concept of unconditional positive regard as a core component of his client-centred therapy, also later known as person-centred counselling. Unconditional positive regard highlights the emphasis this modality has on managing and trying to level power disparities in the consultation room between therapist and client. Developed in the mid-20th century, this therapeutic approach ran counter to the prevailing psycho-analytic and behaviourist paradigms of the time, which could be perceived as pathologising individuals or seemingly redu-cing them to products of their environment. Rogers' humanistic perspective offered a refreshing alternative by emphasising the positive potentials within each person and their capacity for self-actualisation, rather than the therapist as an expert. Person-centred counselling continues to offer a challenge to more pater-nalistic models of mental health care and treatment.

At its core, unconditional positive regard is a fundamental belief in the inherent worth and value of every individual, irre-spective of their actions, behaviours, or characteristics. This concept is grounded in the principles of humanistic psych-ology, emphasising the importance of empathy, acceptance,

DOI: 10.4324/9781003382959-6

and understanding in fostering personal development and psychological well-being. Unconditional positive regard is intricately woven into Rogers' person-centred theory, which posits that individuals naturally strive for personal growth and self-improvement. Rogers believed that individuals possess an inherent drive towards self-actualisation, a process of becoming their true self and reaching their full potential. To facilitate this journey, therapists, educators, and individuals in close relationships must offer unconditional positive regard in order to create an environment where authenticity, vulnerability, and growth can flourish.

What mattered most for Rogers was the relationship a therapist had with their client, with the chances for psychological change enhanced if this relationship met the following six conditions:

1. Two persons are in psychological contact.
2. The first, whom we shall term the client, is in a state of incongruence, being vulnerable or anxious.
3. The second person, whom we shall term the therapist, is congruent or integrated in the relationship.
4. The therapist experiences unconditional positive regard for the client.
5. The therapist experiences an empathic understanding of the client's internal frame of reference and endeavours to communicate this experience to the client.
6. The communication to the client of the therapist's empathic understanding and unconditional positive regard is to a minimal degree achieved.

   No other conditions are necessary. If these six conditions exist, and continue over a period of time, this is sufficient. The process of constructive personality change will follow.

   (Rogers, 1957, p. 96)

Some will further refine these six qualities down to a more essential grouping of numbers 3, 4 and 5. One of three components forming this core of the therapeutic relationship alongside congruence and empathic understanding, unconditional positive regard serves as a cornerstone of client-centred therapy, where therapists create a safe and non-judgemental space for clients to explore their thoughts, emotions and experiences. By providing unconditional positive regard, therapists allow clients to confront their challenges without fear of rejection, enabling them to tap into their inner resources and find relief from that which might be troubling them.

In this chapter, I am conscious that I have focussed more directly on unconditional positive regard instead of empathy – the capacity to understand what might be going on in the client's mind and their subjective experience of the work, and congruence – the therapist's authenticity and genuineness in the therapeutic relationship. Congruence is predicated on a high level of self-awareness to be truly in touch with all aspects of ourselves including those more challenging parts and empathy dependent on being sensitive to that constantly changing flow of experiences coming from the client. Both this form of self-awareness and focussed attention might be more effectively developed from a general meditation technique such as that used to *establish the meditation frame* and also those practices described in the next chapter on Mentalisation-Based Therapy – *The Mentalisation Stance*. However, the meditation method proposed in this chapter will also develop these factors as well.

Rogers' description of unconditional positive regard in his highly influential book *On Becoming A Person* clearly defines the different aspects of unconditionality, positivity and how this is communicated to a client through an attitude that the therapist embodies rather than a specific technique:

> When the therapist is experiencing a warm, positive and acceptant attitude toward what is in the client, this facilitates change. It involves the therapist's genuine willingness for the client to be whatever feeling is going on in him at that moment, – fear, confusion, pain, pride, anger, hatred, love, courage, or awe. It means that the therapist cares for the client, in a nonpossessive way. It means that he prizes the client in a total rather than a conditional

way. By this I mean that he does not simply accept the client when he is behaving in certain ways, and disapprove of him when he behaves in other ways. It means an outgoing positive feeling without reservations, without evaluations. The term we have come to use for this is unconditional positive regard.

(Rogers, 1961, p. 65)

Brian Thorne, emeritus professor of counselling and person-centred counsellor, further emphasises this aspect of acceptance as fully taking into account the full spectrum of a client's being:

Rogers' concept of acceptance of which the term 'unconditional positive regard' is an elaboration, implies a caring by the therapist which is totally uncontaminated by judgements or evaluations of the thoughts, feelings or behaviour of the client. The therapist does not accept some aspects of the client and reject others. He or she experiences (and this cannot be simulated) an outgoing, positive, non-possessive warmth for the client. Such acceptance extends to the full range of the client's feelings and attitudes, from hostility and indifference to love and joy.

(Thorne, 2003, pp. 37–38)

David Mearns, professor of counselling and person-centred therapist, describes a common misconception of unconditional positive regard where it can be downplayed as similar to simply liking, but rather is a significant undertaking for a therapist to develop:

… it involves the counsellor in considerable personal development work to attain a level of personal security and self-acceptance which reduces her need to protect self against others. Unless that extensive personal development work takes place any 'display' of unconditional positive regard on the part of the counsellor tends to be superficial and usually wilts under the challenge of well-developed client self-protective systems. Indeed, this superficial portrayal of unconditional positive regard is usually no better than 'liking' in that it is highly selective: the counsellor finds it possible to portray it towards certain clients who exhibit a similarity of values, but not to others who are different from her.

(Mearns, 2003, p.4)

That is why meditation can be a powerful adjunct in the development of this capacity, given that clients are often acutely sensitive to any approach or intervention which might be more of a *display* than one informed by authenticity and fully embodied by the therapist. Rogers' (1980) description of the therapeutic presence, as exemplified by unconditional positive regard, empathic understanding and congruence, was as he named his 1980 book – *A Way of Being*. Much like meditation, the capacity to develop unconditional positive regard is not one learned from a book or during academic seminars but rather in practical methods of self-discovery and development. While personal therapy, experiential groups, clinical work and other opportunities to be present with someone in a caring capacity can serve this function, meditation also offers this space.

In the method described below, we will express our unconditional positive regard between different groups visualised in our mind's eye. Movement between the different stages where it will first be expressed to ourselves, people close to us and clients with whom we may have had more challenging relationships helps to develop an understanding through experience rather than intellectual understanding. This allows for a less selective and more in-depth developmental process to steer away from that superficial *liking* about which Mearns warns towards a full position for which Rogers advocates.

One small study involving therapists training in person-centred counselling found that practising secular mindfulness meditation practices worked well to help engender unconditional positive regard:

All participants in the study referred to mindfulness complementing and enhancing their understanding of the person-centred therapeutic approach and their own

sense of facilitating presence and of the core conditions
to others and towards themselves.

(Holt, 2022, p. 547)

Therefore, readers might think that the technique for
establishing the meditation frame would be sufficient. However,
I feel that the following method might run closer to specifically developing the mindset of unconditional positive regard
instead of a general therapeutic mindset that might slot into this
approach. The meditation exercise proposed below is one that has
been adapted from a Buddhist practice which seeks to develop
and use as a focus of concentration the emotional experience of
goodwill or loving-kindness. Many people use it as their main
form of meditation as it both offers a strong focus for developing
concentration and also one of personal emotional development
as the generation of these states of goodwill can then translate
off the meditation cushion into everyday life. It can also feel quite
pleasant during and after practicing bringing joy and compassion into the forefront of one's life, which can make it easier to
commit to a regular practice. A similar practice may be known
to readers from its clinical application for clients in some of the
third wave cognitive behaviour therapy (CBT) modalities that
incorporate various compassion focussed mindfulness meditation techniques. Practitioners of these modalities are encouraged
to practice those mindfulness practices which are taught and
used within the therapeutic process by clients.

A certain level of theoretical and practical understanding of
unconditional positive regard is needed as a prerequisite to the
technique. In essence understanding, especially as an emotional
experience, can be used as a springboard to start directing unconditional positive regard towards different objects and then eventually simply as an experience in and of itself. That might seem a
bit of a double bind – an expectation to know something before
developing it, but it is something that will inevitably emerge
from established training methods – being in therapy, practising
clinically, supervising and learning from other's clinical work as
well as through a meditation practice such as the one expounded
below.

Meditation Exercise – Developing Unconditional Positive Regard

Before beginning the exercise, it is necessary to imagine three different categories of people which will be focussed on consecutively. The first is someone for who it is easy to feel unconditional positive regard towards. Depending on your level of clinical experience, this could be a client who you have found it particularly easy to experience unconditional positive regard or perhaps a family member or close friend. The second is a client or person in your life that you feel relatively neutral towards, whereby it is neither easy nor difficult to feel unconditional positive regard. The third would be a challenging client or someone in your life who, on balance, might stir up more feelings of anger, fear or dislike than those encompassing that of unconditional positive regard. Once you have thought of these three people make sure that you can recall them as needed.

After having established the meditation framework, take your attention from your breath and bring into your mind's eye the first person, that is, the person or client it is easy to feel unconditional positive regard towards. See if you can generate some unconditional positive regard towards them, focussing especially on how it feels emotionally, but also any associated physical experience. This is most commonly felt in the chest close to the heart, in the throat area or behind the eyes, but it might also be in the head, hands or really anywhere in which you can notice an association. Try to dwell in that affective and physical experience while keeping the image of the person firmly located in your imagination. Whenever your mind wanders, then mindfully return to the meditation object and continue from there. As always, return to the object with a smile and, in this practice, with the attitude of unconditional positive regard which you are projecting towards the initial person see if you can imagine turning that inwards so that any trace of annoyance with yourself because of mind wandering or physical pains is exposed to the unconditional positive regard.

After at least a few minutes, move on to the second person or client you had thought of, the person whom you feel neutral towards and replace the first person with them in your imagination, continuing to generate that experience of unconditional positive regard noticing the experience both emotionally and physically. Continue this for at least a few more minutes before replacing them with the person or client whom you might find it more challenging to experience unconditional positive regard. If the visualisation breaks down or feels too challenging at any step, then feel free to go back to the person where it feels more comfortable. The purpose of the technique is less about moving through the stages but loosening the connection between a specific person who you might already have an opinion about and the ability to generate unconditional positive regard.

Therefore, having stayed with the third person for a few more minutes, then take that last person from your mind's eye and really focus on just the experience of unconditional positive regard. Try to dwell in whatever degree of unconditional positive regard you have generated and in what is hopefully a pleasant and enjoyable experience. See if you can extend that experience outwards by incorporating not just the three people you have thought of but yourself and anyone else within your circle of friends, family, colleagues and acquaintances and beyond. You can visualise this by imagining this larger group of people surrounding you and being enveloped in your unconditional positive regard radiating from you. Alternatively, or at the same time, you can focus on extending the physical experience of unconditional positive regard spreading within your body beyond that initial place found before and even visualise that radiating from your body as a light or a spreading, shining sensation. See if you can dwell on this experience and stay there for a few minutes more until you are ready to return your attention back to the room.

Some questions on which you could reflect:

◆ Could you notice any differences as you progressed through the different stages of the visualisation?
◆ Did you manage to get a sense of what unconditional positive regard feels like emotionally and physically?

◆ How are you feeling after this meditation?
◆ Did you find this focus on a more affective experience easier to focus on or more challenging than other more physical or cognitive-based techniques?

Chapter Summary

◆ Unconditional positive regard alongside empathic understanding and congruence is one of the cornerstones of person-centred counselling
◆ Accessing this mindset can be enhanced by practising a meditation practice that uses a visualisation exercise to bring about feelings of unconditional positive regard to different groups
◆ A focus on the bodily alongside emotional experience helps it to become more readily available in the consultation room.

References

Holt, E. (2022). Student counsellors' experiences of mindfulness as a component of their person-centred counselling training: An interpretative phenomenological analysis. *Counselling and Psychotherapy Research*, 23(2), pp.540–550.

Mearns, D. (2003). *Developing Person-Centred Counselling*, 2nd Edition. London: Sage.

Rogers, C.R. (1957). The necessary and sufficient conditions of therapeutic personality change. *Journal of Consulting Psychology*, 21(2), pp.95–103.

Rogers, C.R. (1961). *On Becoming a Person*. Boston: Houghton Mifflin.

Rogers, C.R. (1980). *A Way of Being*. Boston: Houghton Mifflin.

Thorne, B. (2003). *Carl Rogers*, 2nd Edition. London: Sage.

7 Existential Psychotherapy
Working Phenomenologically

Existential Psychotherapy

Existential psychotherapy is a philosophical and psychological approach addressing the human condition and the challenges individuals face in finding meaning and purpose in their lives. Differing from other therapeutic modalities, which generally find their roots in psychiatry or psychology, existential psychotherapy has its foundations in existential philosophy. Philosophers including Søren Kierkegaard, Friedrich Nietzsche, Jean-Paul Sartre, Martin Heidegger and Albert Camus all explored fundamental aspects of human existence upon which existential psychotherapy is based, including freedom, responsibility, mortality, isolation and the search for meaning. Existential psychotherapy is not a specific set of techniques but rather a way of understanding and working with clients that emphasises their unique subjective experiences and the choices they make in the face of life's uncertainties. As such, the therapist occupies an existential attitude from where they can be open to supporting the client to reach a place of more understanding and meaning in their lives to manage the struggles and symptoms which they might bring to therapy. This is developed not only through the various training methods that most therapeutic modalities include, none more important than a therapist's personal therapy, but also through the experience and deep engagement which the therapist has with their own lives.

DOI: 10.4324/9781003382959-7

Like person-centred counselling, existential psychotherapy emerged in the mid-20th century as a response to the prevailing psychoanalytic and behaviourist paradigms. The existential approach also comes from the position of the client being the one who dictates the direction of the therapy, positioning the client as their own expert, already holding the means by which they can understand themselves. The process of both therapies allow clients to rediscover their own beliefs and values to bring meaning and authenticity to their lives. They also both hold a phenomenological orientation, that every individual has their own subjective experience of reality, requiring the therapist to enter this reality without the therapist's own presuppositions that may distort this understanding. It is this phenomenological aspect of existential psychotherapy which we will delve into further, offering an opportunity for a meditation method to investigate and develop this attitude and mindset.

Well-known figures in the development of existential psychotherapy include Viktor Frankl, Rollo May, and Irvin Yalom. Frankl (1905–1997) was an Austrian psychiatrist who emphasised the importance of man's will to meaning in all circumstances as a central motivational force, even in the face of profound suffering. Frankl developed his school of logotherapy building on his experiences in Nazi concentration camps (Frankl, 1946). Rollo May (1909–1994) was an American existential psychologist who, drawing on existential philosophy, explored the role of anxiety and the human struggle for authenticity (May, 1969). Irvin Yalom, a contemporary American existential psychiatrist, is known for his work on existential group therapy and accounts of his clinical work written for lay as well as professional audiences (Yalom, 1989). Yalom focusses on the interpersonal dynamics of existential issues, including death, freedom, isolation and meaning (Yalom, 1980).

Just as with other therapies, the existential approach encompasses many of the same common factors, such as presence and authenticity previously mentioned as well as an overlap with the more specific stances explored in the psychoanalytic and person-centred chapters. For this reason, working phenomenologically has been selected for further investigation as it represents an important aspect specific to this therapeutic modality and can provide perspectives on meditation methods that have not been covered elsewhere in this book.

Phenomenology

Phenomenology concerns itself with the study of phenomena, a word derived from the Greek *phainomenon* meaning *things appearing in view*. It is, therefore, concerned with how things appear to be or are experienced and presented to our consciousness. Edmund Husserl (1859–1938) was an Austrian-German mathematician and philosopher who established the school of phenomenology. Through the process of phenomenological, eidetic and transcendental reductions, he attempted to develop a scientific basis for this strand of philosophy to peel away layers of symbolism and so reduce phenomena to their most essential qualities. Husserl (1925) believed that this form of psychology would be the beginning of a rethinking and a starting point for all sciences. Such is the centrality of the phenomenological approach in existential psychotherapy, the existential psychotherapist Ernesto Spinelli prefers the nomenclature of *phenomenological psychotherapy* with the phenomenological enquiry forming a mainstay in terms of therapeutic technique:

> The existential psychotherapist's task centres upon a number of fundamental attitudes that are derived from phenomenological inquiry. In brief, these require the therapist to make the attempt to
>
> 1. Set aside, or bracket, his or her own beliefs, theories, biases and assumptions;
> 2. Emphasize and explore the client's immediate conscious experience of 'being-with-another' (the therapist);
> 3. Focus the investigation upon its descriptive components rather than rely upon theory-driven interpretations.
>
> (Spinelli, 2005, p. 146)

This enquiry is extended through a process known as reductions of experiences. We will be guided by Emmy van Deurzen, a Dutch existential psychotherapist working and teaching in London, UK, through these three stages of reduction, incorporating some of Husserl's more technical language remaining in the original German. The reductions allow the therapist to occupy a position that can get in touch with a more refined state of mind which in turn can create a specific intersubjective experience in the consultation room.

> The objective of existential therapy is for the therapist to purify their consciousness as much as possible and to show how this can be done. This provides an experiential model of connectivity and understanding for the client that will encourage them to do the same from where they stand. It will also lead to moments where therapist and client connect in a surprising and very special sense of togetherness that is that of lived inter-subjectivity.
>
> (van Deurzen and Adams, 2016, p. 169)

Using Husserl's more technical language, the phenomenological reduction is concerned with the process (noesis or cogitatio) of consciousness, the eidetic reduction with the object (noemata or cogitations) of consciousness and the transcendental reduction with the subject (nous or cogito) of consciousness (van Deurzen, 2014).

Phenomenological Reduction

The position of the therapist, their attitude and mindset as with the other therapy modalities in this book is central to existential psychotherapy and it is from here that the phenomenological enquiry can proceed. The phenomenological reduction monitors the process of interaction between therapist and client and involves:

1. The Noesis: focusing on the process of awareness.
2. Epoché: suspending assumptions.
3. Description rather than interpretation.

4. Equalization: having an open mind and balanced attention.
5. Horizontalization: awareness of context and perspective.
6. Verification: returning to actual experience to check our findings again and again.

(van Deurzen and Adams, 2016, pp. 141–142)

The awareness of processes, or noesis, can be brought about during the *Establishing the Meditation Frame* a method by which the reader will now be familiar. This mindset can then be brought to an increased focus on assumptions the therapist might have. They encompass a range of criteria which van Deurzen and Adams (2016, p.48) classify as:

◆   *Physical assumptions* like: "My children will not die before me."
◆   *Social assumptions* like: "Other people are a lot of trouble."
◆   *Psychological assumptions* like: "I never get to do things the way I want."
◆   *Spiritual/ethical assumptions* like: "People should be punished if they do bad things."

The bracketing of the therapist's own beliefs that follows, also known as the rule of epoché, is an aspirational quality that can never be completely fulfilled. It represents an attempt to embody a position open-minded enough to base any conclusions about the client on a more immediate experience instead of one informed by one's own biases and expectations. Prejudices and assumptions are noted and consciously put to one side simply through the process of becoming aware of one's perspective. It is a place of non-judgemental rather than evaluating discernment.

Descriptions are made in a repeated fashion of the phenomena under observation rather than an interpretation. This aims to arrive at a description which is as close to the true nature of the phenomena as possible. Next, we find the process of equalising by not privileging any particular aspect of the phenomena over another. With horizontalising, everything is put into a wider context and the environment that affects the phenomena is considered. Attitudes such as empathy as well as other biases are suspended to remove prejudices and conclusions previously drawn. Once again, it is not possible to fully know the context or full picture of another's experience, but the efforts keep the therapist in a position of not-knowing, questioning and withholding the imposition of assumptions onto the other's subjective experience.

Lastly, we come to verification. This involves the checking in that observations correlate with reality and that the description is accurate. The aim is for verification to help explore meaning. In therapy this involves checking in with a client about how closely their experience matches the descriptions that the therapist is providing. In an internal mindset, this is accomplished through the functions of alertness – monitoring the present moment, as well as ardency – working towards a position of closer connection between subjective and objective experiences while dropping the assumptions that can obscure this.

Spinelli (2005) simplifies the phenomenological reduction into three steps:

A. The Rule of Epoché
B. The Rule of Description
C. The Rule of Horizontalisation/Equalisation

These steps he describes as *points of focus* so as not to treat them as needing to occur consequentially or completely fulfilled in turn. They can provide steps upon which our meditation method is based.

After the phenomenological reduction, two further reductions – eidetic and transcendental can follow. Each brings more focus – eidetic to the objects of consciousness in a similar way to the phenomenological reduction and transcendental to our own subjective participation as the subject of consciousness (van Deurzen, 2011 pp. 41–42).

Eidetic Reduction

The eidetic reduction focusses in on the study of essences in order to identify the more basic building blocks of the phenomena, of the objects of consciousness. There is an imagining or visualisation of the object, a varying of its features and observing if the object still retains its essence. If the facet which has been changed still allows for the survival of the object, then it is inessential to the essence. The French philosopher Descartes' (1596–1650) wax argument is an example of this reduction. Descartes considers the various physical properties of wax as it moves closer to a fire in his *Meditation II – Of the Nature of the Human Mind; and that it is more easily known than the Body*:

> Perhaps it was what I now think, viz. that this wax was not that sweetness of honey, nor that agreeable scent of flowers, nor that particular whiteness, nor that figure, nor that sound, but simply a body which a little while before appeared to me as perceptible under these forms, and which is now perceptible under others. But what, precisely, is it that I imagine when I form such conceptions? Let us attentively consider this, and, abstracting from all that does not belong to the wax, let us see what remains. Certainly nothing remains excepting a certain extended thing which is flexible and movable.
>
> (Descartes, 1911, pp. 414–415)

Therefore, Descartes reaches those more essential characteristics of wax as *a certain extended thing which is flexible and movable*, when before it had melted perhaps shape, scent or colour might have seemed to be intrinsic. Once those aspects had changed, he still considered the material left to be wax. A Cartesian approach might not resonate with all existential psychotherapists and philosophers. Descartes' most famous principle of *cogito, ergo sum* (I think therefore I am), is a source of much debate, such as by Jean-Paul Sartre (1905–1980), a French existential philosopher. Sartre came from an approach where consciousness is embodied, and experience precedes essence. In addition, Martin Heidegger (1889–1976) a German existential and phenomenological philosopher bringing in an emphasis on the awareness of mortality in his counter to Descartes' principle as *I myself am in that I will die* (Heidegger, 1992, p. 316). However, I find Descartes' wax metaphor to be helpful in illustrating the eidetic reduction. Also, this is not the place to be delve into the various philosophical debates and strands associated with existential psychotherapy, but I thought it important to mention this division.

As with the phenomenological reduction, the eidetic reduction can go through a process considering:

1. The Noema: focusing the objects of our awareness.
2. Things come to us under different aspects: profiles, adumbrations or Abschattungen.
3. We tune into our intuitive grasp of things, by the Wesenschau: the seeing of essences.
4. We remember that things are genetically constituted. They are not static but dynamic and change over time.
5. We look for universals beyond the apparent properties and qualities of something.

(van Deurzen and Adams, 2016, p. 142)

There is a reduction as the perception of the objects are denuded of their inessential characteristics and there is an engagement with these more refined aspects in a more direct relationship.

Transcendental Reduction

The third reduction might be one which holds more familiar language to the process of meditation, especially because of the widely practised Transcendental Meditation mantra-based meditation tradition made most famous by The Beatles and its founder Maharishi Mahesh Yogi. The transcending aspect of both these approaches is that beyond the mundane, beyond the everyday self and to something greater than the usual way of relating with the world, others and ourselves. The transcendental reduction brings attention towards a more pure awareness beyond one's own character, psychology and assumptions. It is an awareness that can brings us to a more connected mindset where the divisions between ourselves and others are reduced due to making contact with this transcendental ego – the cogito in Husserl's nomenclature. There is an awareness of the limits when the position of the perspective through which all phenomena are perceived is solely from the self's position. A perspective that might alter this position is reached through a transcendent intersubjectivity - the perspective of being able to experience the connections between our perspectives others' perspectives and the fusion of these to create a wider awareness. The steps are summed up by van Deurzen and Adams (2016, pp. 168–169) as follows:

1. It is about focusing on the cogito, or the consciousness of the thinking self.

2. It seeks to reach towards the transcendental ego; that is, the thinking self rather than the characteristics of the ego that we put forward into social situations.

3. When we turn to our consciousness as a source of understanding and clarity we are not being selfish or ego-centric or solipsistic. On the contrary, we are going to a place where we connect with other people's own pure transcendental consciousness and overcome the separation of our varied world situations.

4. We become aware of our own limits when we do this, as we can never look beyond the horizon of our intentionality. We realize that we cannot look over the horizon unless we move to a different position.

5. Whatever we do and however much we can put ourselves in other people's shoes, the reality remains that our consciousness is always centred around itself. Our self remains the point zero of all our experience.

6. When we do try to stand beyond our normal position of a biased worldview, we begin to translate human experience into a lingua franca, from where we can start to understand different points of view. This is what Husserl called 'transcendental inter-subjectivity', because we connect with other people in a new way.

Van Deurzen offers a compelling example of *doing phenomenology* through a reflective exercise with the natural surroundings as the objects of experience (van Deurzen, 2011, pp. 42–43). Van Deurzen is able to connect with her natural surroundings through each reduction changing her relationship with the world through these phenomenological reductions. In order to create a meditation method of reflection relevant to clinical practice, we will take the object of experience as a clinical session or client first brought into the mind.

Meditation Exercise – A Phenomenological Reflection

After having *Established The Meditation Frame*, bring into the mind's eye a client or specific session with that client. Imagine their physical presence – what they look like, their physical mannerisms and how they were in relation to you. This will require quite a focussed awareness which is evaluating as you distinguish what is useful to put effort into bringing into your imagination. Employ ardency to build the picture up and alertness to notice what it might look and feel like. Bring into the mind your emotional responses to the client before, during and after the session. Bring to mind some of the things you both said and the impact it had on both of you. Try to get a sense of their presence in the physical, affective and cognitive realms.

Once the image of the client or session is firmly in your mind, we can turn to the phenomenological reduction. See if you can identify and then bracket any assumptions that arise for you about the client both surfacing now and those which you might have generated in an effort to bring them into your mind. Open up your awareness and employ a non-judgemental discernment to whatever perceptions might be arising. Notice what might be coming up as you keep the client within your awareness. You will inevitably start employing descriptions, making them as objective as possible within imposing assumptions through interpretation. Do not privilege one phenomenon over another, keeping equalisation in mind. As impressions continue to become apparent, see if you can widen your perception of the client beyond their current manifestation, becoming aware of their intercultural context and personal history. Continue to bracket any assumptions that occur and follow the rules of epoché, description, horizontalisation and equalisation. As the awareness becomes broader and your perception of the client becomes more open to different meanings, moving away from your own preconceptions and assumptions, we can approach the eidetic reduction.

Making this mindset more stripped of those features of assumptions, the eidetic reduction takes us closer to the essence of the client and what they are bringing to the therapy. Bring in a sense of wonder and curiosity as to what this person might be like or how the session was. Take note of what comes to mind with regards to the client or the session, see if you remove this from your impression to see if it is inessential to their essence. Try to refine and strip away the image you have of what constitutes the most essential aspects of their being. See if you can find what lies behind the client, behind the language they use, the defences they might employ, their physicality and the more everyday way of relating that might come into sessions. Notice how many of these characteristics, even those that appear the most integral are in flux and constant change both throughout the life of the client, in between sessions and even within the different moments of the session. Take as broad a view as possible of this person, are there elements of their being that you can reach which are common to yourself or even all humanity?

Now come to the transcendental reduction. Allow the image of the client or session to melt away in your mind's eye. At the same time, see if you can turn your awareness to the part of the mind that seems to have been observing and noticing, the place within the mind from which self-awareness sits. Any time a perception of the self arises, see if you can bring your attention to the transcendental ego – the focus of consciousness instead of personal perspective. Try to map out this sense of awareness, the limits of the connections it might have with others as well as the centre from which this experience of consciousness emerges. Be aware that these may not have a geographical location, or if they do, that this might not necessarily be in the area of the head. Appreciate the commonality of this consciousness and the profound appreciation of this awareness of awareness that can bring so much meaning to our existence. Dwell in this expansive sense of consciousness before emerging from the meditation.

Some questions on which you could reflect:

◆ Could you notice the different qualities of experience between the different reductions?
◆ Did it feel quite mechanistic at times, or were you able to flow between the different levels of the reductions?
◆ How do you feel emerging from the transcendental aspect of the meditation?
◆ When returning to the theoretical aspects of phenomenology, has the meditation added any depth of meaning through experience?

Chapter Summary

◆ The phenomenological approach offers a unique perspective on the therapeutic encounter
◆ By following phenomenological, eidetic and transcendental reductions, therapists can get to a more essential focus in the consultation room
◆ Using a visualisation meditation method, bringing in a specific client or session can develop a phenomenological approach to understanding the therapeutic relationship.

References

Descartes, R. (1911). *The Philosophical Works of Descartes* (1970), trans. E. S. Haldane. Cambridge: Cambridge University Press.

Frankl, V.E. (1946). *Man's Search for Meaning*. Boston: Beacon Press.

Heidegger, M. (1992). *History of the Concept of Time: Prolegomena*. Bloomington: Indiana University Press.

Husserl, E. (1925) *Phenomenological Psychology* (1977). trans. J. Scanlon. The Hague: Martinus Nijhoff.

May, R. (1969). *Love and Will*. New York: W.W. Norton.

Spinelli, E. (2005). *The Interpreted World: An Introduction to Phenomenological Psychology*, 2nd Edition. Los Angeles: Sage.

van Deurzen, E. (2011). *Everyday Mysteries: A Handbook of Existential Psychotherapy*, 2nd Edition. London; New York: Routledge.

van Deurzen, E. (2014). Structural existential analysis (SEA): A phenomenological method for therapeutic work. *Journal of Contemporary Psychotherapy*, 45(1), pp.59–68.

van Deurzen, E. and Adams, M. (2016). *Skills in Existential Counselling & Psychotherapy*. Los Angeles: Sage.

Yalom, I.D. (1980). *Existential Psychotherapy*. New York: Basic Books.

Yalom, I.D. (1989). *Love's Executioner and Other Tales of Psychotherapy*. London, England: Penguin Books.

8 Mentalisation-Based Therapy

The Mentalising Stance

Mentalisation-based therapy (MBT) is a psychotherapy modality developed by Peter Fonagy – a Hungarian-born British psychoanalyst and clinical psychologist, with Anthony Bateman – a British psychiatrist and psychotherapist. It was initially developed in the early 2000s for borderline personality disorder and has now been adapted for a wider range of mental health issues, including other personality disorders, eating disorders, depression, trauma and drug addiction. MBT is designed for clients who might experience intense emotional distress that can be overwhelming and are prone to destructive behaviours towards themselves or others. It is also directed towards people who are distrustful of others and might find it hard to understand other people's responses to them. Unlike the other psychotherapy modalities in this book, which are not time-limited or manualised, MBT is a manualised therapy which usually lasts for 12–18 months and is usually delivered as both group and one-on-one therapy simultaneously.

First, it is important to establish what mentalising is:

> Mentalization, or better mentalizing, is the process by which we make sense of each other and ourselves, implicitly and explicitly, in terms of subjective states and mental processes. It is a profoundly social construct in the sense

DOI: 10.4324/9781003382959-8

that we are attentive to the mental states of those we are with, physically or psychologically. Given the generality of this definition, most mental disorders will inevitably involve some difficulties with mentalization. In fact, we can conceive of most mental disorder as the mind misinterpreting its own experience of itself, thus ultimately a disorder of mentalization. However, the key issue is whether the dysfunction is core to the disorder and/or a focus on mentalization is heuristically valid, i.e. provides an appropriate domain for therapeutic intervention.

(Bateman and Fonagy, 2010, p. 12)

Mentalisation is also often summarised by the simpler definitions of *understanding misunderstanding* or *thinking about thinking*. Change in MBT occurs through a focus on the mentalising process combined with an increase in epistemic trust. This epistemic trust is triggered by a client being with a therapist who can give them an experience of being understood on their own terms. This allows for a relaxing of vigilance and suspicion towards a willingness to accept new knowledge or another as trustworthy and being able to generalise this to other people and situations. There is the development of a greater capacity for mentalising through a safe attachment relationship with the therapist where the client can feel able to explore the mind of another.

The Mentalising Stance

The mindset of the therapist is orientated around a concept called the *mentalising stance*:

We advocate maintaining a mentalizing stance as providing the best chance of achieving mentalizing goals. That is, in conducting psychotherapy, we strive to maintain an inquisitively curious, not-knowing attitude—which requires tolerance for ambiguity and uncertainty in the therapist, just as the mentalizing stance requires of patients.

(Allen, Fonagy and Bateman, 2008, p. 182)

The mentalisation stance in MBT refers to the therapist's approach and mindset when engaging with a client. Some of the elements will be familiar as common factors described earlier in the book. However, the mentalisation stance encompasses a more specific mindset involving the therapist's ability to understand, interpret, and respond to both their own and the client's thoughts, feelings, and intentions. This stance is rooted in empathy, curiosity, and a genuine desire to comprehend the client's inner world, as well as a focus on the therapist's capacity for mentalising. It includes a range of characteristics mentioned in the following subsections.

Empathetic Curiosity

Therapists aim to genuinely understand the client's perspective without judgement or preconceived notions. They recognise that clients' behaviours, emotions, and thoughts are often shaped by underlying experiences and beliefs. By approaching the client with genuine curiosity, therapists create an environment where the client feels valued, heard, and encouraged to explore their thoughts and feelings more openly. This can help to foster epistemic trust.

Reflective Inquiry

Therapists engage in reflective inquiry, actively seeking to uncover the meaning behind the client's words and actions. Rather than making assumptions, they remain non-judgemental and ask open-ended questions, inviting clients to reflect on their experiences, motivations, and emotions. This approach encourages clients to delve deeper into their inner world, fostering self-awareness and insight.

Avoiding Assumptions

There is an avoidance of making and bracketing of assumptions about the client's thoughts and feelings. Therapists understand that their own biases, past experiences, and cultural backgrounds can influence their interpretations, so are put to one side. Instead of making any premature conclusions, therapists remain open to multiple interpretations and are willing to validate the client's experiences, even if they differ from their own.

Promoting Secure Attachment

A safe and supportive environment allow clients to explore their emotions and thoughts, reducing fears of judgement. This secure attachment fosters epistemic trust, enabling clients to share their vulnerabilities and challenges more openly.

Cultivating Mindful Presence

The mentalisation stance requires therapists to be fully present and attuned during sessions according to the definition of mindfulness as per MBSR and MBCT. Mindful presence in MBT involves being in the moment, actively listening, and picking up on verbal and nonverbal cues from the client. This level of attentiveness allows therapists to accurately perceive the client's emotions and thoughts, enhancing their ability to respond empathetically and effectively.

Navigating Ambiguity

As human experiences are often complex and ambiguous, mentalisation-based therapists acknowledge that clients' emotions and thoughts can be multifaceted and may not have straightforward explanations. Instead of coming from a solutions-focussed perspective, therapists explore the nuances of the client's experiences, helping them make sense of their internal conflicts.

Fostering Collaboration

MBT is a collaborative endeavour. Therapists partner with clients to co-create insights and strategies for growth. By involving clients in the process of exploring their inner world, therapists empower them to take an active role.

Modelling Mentalisation

By demonstrating mentalisation as the ability to consider various perspectives, including that of the other, therapists encourage clients to develop their own mentalisation skills. Clients learn not only how to understand themselves better but also how to navigate their relationships outside the therapy room.

Managing Countertransference

Therapists reflect on their emotional responses to understand how these responses might be connected to the client's experiences. This self-awareness helps therapists maintain objectivity and ensure that their reactions do not hinder the therapeutic process. Being in touch with and processing countertransference also helps to develop robustness.

Following on from these characteristics, while it is important for the therapist to maintain a level of robustness and resilience, they must also be able to recognise when there might be a breakdown in mentalising. This is especially relevant as MBT was first developed to work with populations who had been diagnosed with borderline personality disorder (also known as emotionally unstable or emotional intensity disorder). Resilience is crucial to manage the challenges of working with client populations that may often be overwhelmed by their own distress. This distress can be difficult to contain for the therapist, too and may also result in challenging behaviours that can disrupt the therapeutic relationship and the ability for the therapist to maintain a mentalising stance. It can be especially hard to bear breakdowns when clients struggle to hold onto what is good or might be going well.

This is especially pertinent when working in a group setting. There are many projections coming from different directions with clients, often relating to the therapist as a part object. There can be much anger can be directed at the therapist facilitating the group. Pressure is increased as the therapist has to manage the boundaries of confidentiality, as may be seeing some of the clients on a one-to-one basis. In addition, there can be the very raw experience of envy as clients are faced with having to share their therapist when they may be used to having the therapist's full attention. In contrast with some approaches where the therapist does not share what might be going on in their mind with the client, the therapist shares their own mentalising process even when things break down for themselves. When there are points at which it is not possible for the client or therapist to mentalise, the therapist is expected to realise this has occurred, point it out and recover a mentalising capacity.

The patient may suddenly lose their mentalizing capacity in a session. This may be exampled in many ways, for example by an affect storm, excessive anxiety, sudden change in emotional states. The therapist needs to be able to identify these states of mind rapidly and decrease the level of arousal. Initially this is done by the therapist taking responsibility for triggering the sudden loss of mentalizing in the patient. The therapist explores openly what he might have said or not said, was it the tone of voice, the use of a particular word that might have been the cause of the problem. He refrains from asking the patient to do more therapeutic work at a time when they do not have the capacity to do so. This ability to mentalize in the face of high arousal in the session is an important aspect of MBT if only from the perspective that the patient can identify with the process.

At other times the therapist may lose his own capacity to mentalize. The ability to recognize this, as it is happening, is a key skill as is a capacity to regain mentalizing. When loss of mentalizing in the therapist occurs it is necessary to identify the collapse openly with the patient before retracing the session to seek reasons for why it might have occurred. The best position at this point for the MBT therapist is to accept the difficulty – 'I can't think at the moment about this'; 'I am losing the focus of the session' and then to immediately focus on rewinding the session to a point at which both patient and therapist were able to reflect adequately.

(Bateman, Bales and Hutsebaut, 2014, p. 18)

Using those shorter definitions of mentalisation, recovery is facilitated by *understanding the misunderstanding* leading up to a loss of the mentalising capacity by *thinking about the thinking* that did or did not occur. Therapists have to pick the right moment to notice patterns, preventing things becoming too heated, but at the same time, they have to manage themselves to prevent any acting in on the therapist's part. The therapist has to toe a line between interventions designed to engage and help develop a client's ability to mentalise, while also being careful not to cause any harm by overwhelming the client:

> Patients with BPD are sensitive in interpersonal contexts, and particularly vulnerable to deterioration of mental-state awareness in relationships when their poorly organized attachment system is stimulated—as attachment is triggered, mentalizing becomes vulnerable. Combine that with psychotherapy, which is inherently relational, and there is a potentially toxic mix. Consequently, MBT is defined by a constellation of interventions that promote mentalizing, and active avoidance of interventions that might cause harm by undermining mentalizing. The MBT clinician negotiates a potentially stormy passage, balancing attachment stimulation and relational exploration with supporting mentalizing strength. If these two aspects are not balanced so that they work together rather than against each other, patients with BPD will struggle to develop the capacity to function effectively in interpersonal relationships—the lack of which is at the core of their difficulties. Treatment can be effective only if it is able to enhance the patient's mentalizing capacities without generating too many negative (iatrogenic) effects by emotionally overstimulating their attachment system.
>
> (Bateman et al., 2023, p. 44)

Mentalising Imagery Therapy

While researching and developing a visualisation meditation technique to engender the mentalising stance, I came across the work of Felipe Jain, an American psychiatrist. Jain has developed guided imagery and mindfulness techniques to support clients in the development of their own capacity to mentalise. These are based on Buddhist tantra and Upanishadic/Vedantic traditions (Timalsina, 2013) as well as secular mindfulness and imagery rehearsal therapy techniques more often used to treat nightmares secondary to post-traumatic stress disorder (PTSD) (Krakow et al., 2001). The practices specifically support the improved balance between mentalisation and emotional regulation. In two studies, these practices have been combined with an investigation into the dorsolateral prefrontal cortex (DLPFC), which is associated with depression and the regulation of low mood. In addition to improvement in symptoms, it was found that there was increased DLPFC connectivity with an emotion regulation network when these specific meditation techniques were practised for dementia caregivers showing symptoms of depression (Jain et al., 2021, 2022). The adaptability of these practices has allowed them to be customised for a Spanish language remote virtual program delivered to Latino family dementia caregivers (Ramírez-Gomez et al., 2023).

The imagery techniques promote mentalising through four perspectives:

◆ Towards the self from the self – how one views oneself
◆ From others towards the self – how others view oneself
◆ Towards others from the self – how one views others and
◆ From others towards themselves – what others are thinking and feeling themselves.

The methods run through cognitive, affective and embodied realms. Rather than designing entirely new meditation methods given the evidence base already established by Jain's techniques, I have adapted two of the practices – *Nesting Doll* and *Situation Solver* (Jain and Fonagy, 2018) specifically to be used by a therapist in relation to a client, rather than in the more general manner taught to participants in Jain's programs. The emphasis of these practices is on ardency as the instructions propel the meditator through a series of instructions brought to develop a specific visualisation exercise. Alertness connects the meditator to the imagined situation and the developing experience going forward. It is a non-judgemental awareness with both open and focussed features.

Nesting Doll Imagery Practice

The nesting doll imagery practice is a meditation that involves the creation of an imagined model of the self and then another in the centre of the body, enabling you to find a perspective inside yourself and understand others. The visualisation incorporates the embodied self, thoughts, feelings and sense of awareness. It allows you to embrace the fullness of yourself, including negatives and positives as well as the perspectives of another person. In the case of the adapted technique below, that other person is a client. This develops a neutral, non-judgemental point of view towards the self and others allowing for the ambiguity of not knowing and accepting. There is a mindful presence and reflective inquiry as per the mentalising stance. The technique has been adapted from spiritual and religious practices where the meditator seeks to absorb aspects or characteristics of a deity into themselves. In the case of a technique to develop mentalisation, that would be bringing in parts of the self that have been projected out in order to develop a more whole object way of relating to the self and others – that of a progression from paranoid schizoid to depressive position (Klein, 1946). This meditation method helps the practitioners to remember not just their own wholeness but that of others. The end of the meditation encompasses a section on goodwill and compassion in order to cement in this experience by attributing an increased empathic connection to the imagined self and client-other alongside the cognitive, affective and embodied experience already established. It also connects to the development of empathy for self and others described in the mentalising stance. In the next meditation exercise, this nesting doll practice has been adapted to enhance your ability to mentalise in the clinical situation. You will need to think of a particular client, so see if there is a client with whom it might be helpful to get a fuller understanding of their perspective which might currently be obscured or unclear who you can bring to mind.

Meditation Exercise – Developing the Mentalising Stance

After having *Established the Meditation Frame,* visualise a space within the centre of the chest from the front of the body all the way to the back. Physically enlarge this area by broadening your shoulders outwards and extending your spine upwards. Get a sense of the boundaries of this space imagining its walls slightly expanding and contracting with each breath.

Start by forming an imagine of yourself – a nesting doll in this central space. Allow it to contain all your bodily sensations, your thoughts and feelings. Contain within the space that part of you which is observing, listening or reading these instructions and is noticing what is happening now.

Include in the image any movement of the body, that of the body breathing and the subtle movement of the limbs and trunk, which helps the body to balance as well as any movements detected caused by the circulation of blood around the body such as the bobbing of the head or pulsing of limbs in contact with each other. Incorporate into the image all physical sensations, including any pains or tensions that might be present, those more pleasant physical feelings that might have arisen through the process of meditation and the sensations that might have a more neutral quality. Allow all thoughts that arise to be in this image, whether good or bad, helpful or unhelpful or just those neutral descriptors that seemingly occur in the mind completely out of our control. Do the same with emotions, bring them into the nesting doll, anger or happiness, hatred or goodwill and boredom or excitement. Allow them all to exist, arise and pass away together.

Observe all these experiences as part of the whole. Include your identity as a therapist both your internal setting and mindset, the particular approach and techniques which you use and the theoretical underpinning for the modality or multiple models you draw on. Update the doll with the thoughts, feelings, sensations and types of awareness that arise in the here and now.

Now to bring an image of a client into the centre with you. Think about using your perception of them when they're in the consultation room with you, one you find it easier to relate with from a therapeutic stance. First, take a moment to include in the centre your own countertransference in response to the client – how you might experience that in the body, in your thoughts and your feelings. If nothing specific arises, take a moment to just bring in that sense of awareness of the client when you are together in the consultation room.

Now, just as you did with yourself, imagine their own physical experience within their body including their breathing pattern, physical mannerisms, posture and clothing imagining putting that into the model within the space in your chest. Include their thoughts as imagined from their perspective and what feelings they might be experiencing during a session, both positive and more challenging. Include the nature of their awareness which perceives their internal world during sessions with you.

Imagine their transference – their thoughts and feelings towards you. Envision how they experience you in body and mind when you are together, their impression of what you're like and the impact of when they hear what you say. Bring that all together into the central space.

Imagine how your internal stance, interventions and theoretical underpinning of your therapy modality or models therapy manifests in the client's experience of the therapy and how it might impact. Consider how the client experiences the therapeutic process or how they might defend against and resist it. Continue to absorb and contain that into the image in the space you have created.

Now bring both yourself and the client together in the centre. Notice the similarities, that both of you have personal histories and families or other people you grew up with, a range of positive and challenging relationships and all the intercultural backgrounds specific to you and the client. Recognise that you both have kindness with goodwill and also anger within you, that both sides exist together with your own defences and resistances.

With the images of both yourself and the client together, bring up feelings of goodwill and compassion towards them as one in the centre. Use a repeating phrase denoting positive feelings of goodwill if that helps. Just as with the *Developing Unconditional Positive Regard* meditation exercise focus on the physical experience of goodwill and allow it to spread throughout the central space. Extend it to feelings of understanding and acceptance of all the different aspects of yourself and the client which has been brought together.

Allow the image to dissipate and be aware of the space in the centre. Bring your awareness back to the full length of the breath as it is before slowly relaxing and beginning a phase of reflection. Some questions on which to reflect:

- ◆ Could you see how you brought in the four different mentalising perspectives?
- ◆ To what degree was it possible to get in touch with both your own and your client's perspectives and experiences?
- ◆ Do you feel any differently towards your client?
- ◆ Is there any residual awareness in your own body of the visualisation exercise in terms of your physical awareness or emotional experience?
- ◆ Do you feel that your capacity to be able to take a mentalising stance has altered?

Situation Solver Imagery Practice

This practice uses a reflection on a challenging situation that triggered a difficult emotional reaction and behavioural response. It slows down the situation allowing for a space to think about what had occurred to help understand why the situation unfolded as it did. It also includes a section on imagining an alternative ending and how that might come about, similar to how imagery rehearsal therapy may work with imagining and rehearsing alternative endings for nightmares. For the purposes of the adapted technique below, we will use the reflection of a group therapy session, which might be particularly challenging, where mentalising might have broken down for therapist, clients, the whole group or involving an event which did not turn out as wished or expected. I think it is especially helpful to use an event related to when working in a group environment due to the challenges and pressures described above. As with the nesting doll technique, a space in the centre of the body is established where the situation is imagined to occur. It is then replayed imagining how it occurred, incorporating the four different mentalising perspectives outlined above. The broader environmental and historical situation is then brought in, helping to provide a context for the event. It can then be imagined how you might have preferred the situation to have occurred from both the clients', the whole group's and your perspectives. This process helps in the reflection of a situation that might have been overwhelming at the time. While not necessarily literally *solving* the situation, by bringing in other perspectives and meaning to a situation that may be hard to understand, a solution is found in a way through the development and recovery of a mentalising capacity. As a preparation for the exercise, try to think of an event when working in a group setting whereby it might be helpful to develop more of a mentalising stance. If you do not work as a group therapist, then you can adapt this exercise to a specific situation involving one specific client.

Meditation Exercise – Developing and Maintaining Mentalising in Group Work

After practising the *Establishing the Meditation Frame* method, as with the *Adapted Nesting Doll Practice* we begin by creating a psychic space in the centre of the chest. Imagining an empty area that we can physically get in touch with my pulling our shoulders back, taking in a deep breath and extending the spine upwards. Into this space, we will bring the situation on which you wish to reflect. Imagine the event occurring like a play, for the purposes of this exercise, I will assume you have selected a situation in a group setting, but this is not required. Starting from the beginning of the event or session slow things down as much as possible. Focus on the physical situation as well as how it felt for you. Include how your thoughts, feelings and physical experience changed throughout.

In the body, were muscles tensed or clenched, did your breathing change in tempo, depth or quality? Perhaps you were angry, scared, worried, panicked or ashamed. Maybe you felt numb and froze being unsure how to act or what to say. Note any emerging thoughts and fantasies that came up for you. See what your awareness was like, the quality of that part of you which is listening or reading these instructions.

With the event in your central space, see if you can imagine how the clients appeared physically, the impact it had on you and how you imagined their intentions. Can you observe yourself and the clients this time differently, with a calm, accepting and non-judgemental attitude? If not, notice those self-judging voices and how they impact the mind, body and emotional spheres. Can you accept those more uncomfortable emotions and behaviours that the clients displayed and that maybe you responded with. Perhaps you had another therapist co-facilitating the group, include them in the space alongside the clients.

Now we shift to the clients' perspective. Embody the clients involved from head to toe and bring them into the centre. Include their movements when in the room incorporating their physical presence, clothing, mannerisms and breathing. See if you can look through their eyes back at you. Note how you came across them in this situation. Imagine their internal world, their thoughts, feelings in their own body and emotional experiences as they interacted with you and how these change as the situation unfolded. While noticing this, try to calmly accept them, their thoughts and feelings as understandable. If this is not possible, notice those more judging parts in the mind, body and emotional realms.

Return attention to the space at the centre of your body now with both you and them together. Imagine the broader context of the situation. Their past and your past, including early family relationships or the way in which you and them grew up, include the immediate situation for both of you before this event, what both of your environments were like, who else might have been around and the impact on you and them. Imagine those broader intercultural identities which both you and the client bring wherever you might be.

Now imagine how the scenario might have been different, how the situation would have occurred, if you had known the clients' thoughts and feelings and they had known yours. Rehearse a different response. Let the situation unfold if you had brought a state of mind that you would have preferred. Notice the changes in both you and your client's physical response, thoughts and emotions. What went differently in the rehearsal? Even if you feel the outcome didn't change, how did your own experience and that of the client differ? Shift your view back to the client and imagine how they might have experienced you differently, how they might have changed their own reactions as a result and what their own feelings and thoughts about themselves might have been.

Just as with the *Developing The Mentalising Stance* exercise, bring up feelings of goodwill and compassion towards both yourself, the clients and the group as a whole together as one in the central space. Use a repeating phrase denoting positive feelings of goodwill if that helps. Just as with the *Developing Unconditional Positive Regard* meditation exercise focus on the physical experience of goodwill and allow it to spread throughout the central space. Extend it to feelings of understanding and acceptance of all the different aspects of yourself and the clients which have been brought together.

Allow the image to dissipate and be aware of the space in the centre. Bring your awareness back to the full length of the breath as it is before slowly relaxing and beginning a phase of reflection. Some questions on which to reflect:

- ◆ Could you see how you brought in the four different mentalising perspectives?
- ◆ Was it possible to imagine the scenario as well as rehearse an alternative?
- ◆ Do you feel any differently towards your clients or the group as a whole?
- ◆ Now that you have finished the meditation, has your attitude to the situation altered at all?

Chapter Summary

◆ The mentalising stance describes the mindset involved in MBT

◆ By adapting visualisation meditation methods (nesting doll and situation solver techniques) developed for mentalising imagery therapy, it is possible to help enhance the capacity to mentalise in clinical situations

◆ These visualisation exercises can help to develop and maintain mentalising when working with potentially challenging client groups and within group therapy situations.

References

Allen, J.G., Fonagy, P. and Bateman, A. (2008). *Mentalizing in Clinical Practice*. Arlington, Virginie: American Psychiatric Publishing.

Bateman, A., Bales, D. and Hutsebaut, J. (2014). A Quality Manual for MBT. [online] Available at: https://www.annafreud.org/media/1217/a-quality-manual-for-mbt-edited-april-23rd-2014-2.pdf [Accessed 21 October 2023].

Bateman, A. and Fonagy, P. (2010). Mentalization based treatment for borderline personality disorder. *World Psychiatry*, 9(1), pp.11–15.

Bateman, A., Fonagy, P., Campbell, C., Luyten, P. and Debbané, M. (2023). *Cambridge Guide to Mentalization-Based Treatment (MBT)*. Cambridge: Cambridge University Press.

Jain, F.A., Chernyak, S., Nickerson, L., Abrams, M., Iacoboni, M., Christov-Moore, L., Connolly, C.G., Fisher, L.B., Sakurai, H., Bentley, K., Tan, E., Pittman, M., Lavretsky, H. and Leuchter, A.F. (2021). Mentalizing imagery therapy for depressed family dementia caregivers: Feasibility, clinical outcomes and brain connectivity changes. *Journal of Affective Disorders Reports*, 5, p.100–155.

Jain, F.A., Chernyak, S.V., Nickerson, L.D., Morgan, S., Schafer, R., Mischoulon, D., Bernard-Negron, R., Nyer, M., Cusin, C., Ramirez Gomez, L. and Yeung, A. (2022). Four-week mentalizing imagery therapy for family dementia caregivers: A randomized controlled trial with neural circuit changes. *Psychotherapy and Psychosomatics*, 91(3), pp.180–189.

Jain, F.A. and Fonagy, P. (2018). Mentalizing imagery therapy: Theory and case series of imagery and mindfulness techniques to understand self and others. *Mindfulness*, 11(1), pp.153–165.

Klein, M. (1946). Notes on some schizoid mechanisms. *The International Journal of Psycho-Analysis*, 27(Pt 3–4), pp.99–110.

Krakow, B., Hollifield, M., Johnston, L., Koss, M., Schrader, R., Warner, T.D., Tandberg, D., Lauriello, J., McBride, L., Cutchen, L., Cheng, D., Emmons, S., Germain, A., Melendrez, D., Sandoval, D. and Prince, H. (2001). Imagery rehearsal therapy for chronic nightmares in sexual assault survivors with posttraumatic stress disorder. *JAMA*, 286(5), p.537.

Ramírez-Gomez, L., Johnson, J.K., Ritchie, C.S., Meyer, A., Tan, E., Madarasmi, S., Gutierrez-Ramirez, P., Aldarondo-Hernández, C., Mischoulon, D., Banerjee, S. and Jain, F.A. (2023). Virtual mentalizing imagery therapy for Spanish language Latino family dementia caregivers: A feasibility and acceptability study. *Frontiers in Psychology*, 14:961835, pp.01–07.

Timalsina, S. (2013). Imagining reality: Image and visualization in classical Hinduism. *Southeast Review of Asian Studies*, 35, pp.50–69.

9 Other Complementary Techniques

The main thrust of the book has been concerned with the use of meditation as an adjunct to conventional training methods to develop the specific mindsets of various therapy modalities. I would also like to explore some other techniques that may also be useful to complement the practices described. In addition, as I touched on in the introduction, the techniques that I have suggested are not necessarily the definitive types for each mindset mentioned. There are also other psychotherapy modalities that I have not explored with their own perspectives. By the end of the book, perhaps there will be ideas forming for you about which techniques may be most suited to your practice, but also your own specific psyche. Many therapists also work in an eclectic and integrative manner. Therefore, they may bring different modalities and mindsets to a session depending on the client and where the client might be in that particular session or moment of time. For this reason, I wanted to bring in these other practices so that you might find different ways of using meditation in your own work with clients. Meditation is also a fantastic system for personal development and by being aware of a wider range of techniques, there could be a specific way of meditating which works best for you in which you want to delve deeper. For example, seated meditation may not be attractive, given the amount of sitting you might do when speaking with clients. Therefore, a walking meditation might be more helpful for you. It might be challenging for you to close your eyes for longer periods of time, so perhaps meditations involving open

DOI: 10.4324/9781003382959-9

eyes may be more appropriate. Whatever the reason may be, I have presented the following techniques to give a wider range of approaches to accompany the diversity of practitioners out there.

The meditation methods I have proposed to match with specific therapeutic mindsets have been suggested with the understanding that they are worked on outside of the consultation room in an effort to develop the stance, which is then brought to a session. In this chapter, I will make some suggestions about how meditation can be used after sessions to reflect and develop an understanding about a case, in the room with a client and also for preparations before a session.

Box Breathing

This is a simple breathwork exercise, which I have often taught as a means to reduce worry or panic alongside cyclic sighing. However, it can be used in any situation where you wish to introduce some calm and alertness as it brings awareness to the breath, slows it down and focusses attention on the physical environment in a simple and memorable manner. For this reason, it can be thought of as a grounding exercise. At the same time, some people will use box breathing as their main meditation technique, practising it, for example, five minutes a day. It is also taught to people who work in high-stress situations with the most common example quoted for its efficacy as part of US Navy SEAL training.

I like to add in eye movements to introduce a focus on the environment, but you can also perform it with eyes closed, concentrating solely on the breathing without the eye movements included. I think the addition of the eye movement makes it more effective in terms of grounding and gives more for the mind to focus on, especially if it is restless. This makes it a great starting point if the mind is wandering too much to be able to focus enough on the breath or another meditation object. At the same time, as there is less turning inwards it reduces the potential for high levels of focus. It can be practised wherever you might be and no one around needs to know what you might be doing. For this reason, it might be particularly effective, alongside taking a few sighs if, for example, you are feeling anxious before a presentation, interview, or as might occur before seeing a specific client, especially in your early career.

Look around and see if you can see something box-shaped be that a square or rectangle. Any four-sided, two-dimensional shape. This could be a window, the back of your telephone or brick on a wall. Start by looking at the bottom left corner and slowly take a deep breath in, counting to four as you bring your gaze to the top left corner. When arriving there hold your breath as you count up to four once again and look over to the top right corner. Then breathe out completely as you count to four and look to the bottom right corner. Holding your out-breath, without breathing in again, count up to four looking along the bottom of the box back to the bottom left corner before taking a deep breath in and starting the process again.

This can be summarised for these four steps, each lasting four seconds or longer:

1. Breathe in
2. Hold in-breath
3. Breath out
4. Hold out-breath.

Try to increase the number you are counting to or slow the gaps between the numbers, especially if you are feeling worried or panicked. It might be that the first time around the box, you go quite quickly and then on consequential times round, everything slows down. You can also do this exercise, as mentioned before, without looking at a box or without counting at all. Some people also visualise the box in their mind's eye with their eyes closed. You can even download a GIF and use that to guide you. Whichever way you do it, try to practise a few ways to find which is the most effective, but also so that it's in your muscle memory. Then, when you might be feeling especially anxious, you can draw on this simple but effective technique to establish some calm and centre yourself before undertaking whatever activity might be the source of some of the worry.

Walking Meditation

I think walking meditation is an excellent alternative to sitting meditation and by no means any less effective. Due to the movement of the body, it offers a midpoint between sitting and bringing awareness to the body and mind when going about everyday activities. A modified form can also be performed when walking from place to place, for example, on the way to catch a bus or down a long corridor. One hospital I used to work in had an exceptionally long corridor that might take up to five minutes to walk. I often took it as an opportunity to practise walking meditation and create some space in my mind during a long shift. Due to the motion of the body, some people find it easier than when sitting to maintain alertness.

Begin by finding a quiet and peaceful location where you can walk undisturbed. This could be indoors, but given space can be limited, outdoors is also fine, although there can be potentially more distractions in the environment, so it depends if you are able to maintain your focus. You have a choice between either walking to a specific destination, round in a circular motion or more traditionally back and forth in a straight line from one place to another. I will describe an exercise for the latter as it is the way I mostly practise, but find which way is most suitable for you. Walking back and forth outside can be particularly helpful to form a routine as by walking along the same path repeatedly you will form a groove in the earth. If walking on a lawn, you might create a path with an absence of grass. This can then be a visual reminder of your meditation practice and can form a specific relationship between you and that location, which can motivate and tie your practice to that particular path. However, you can also practise in a similar way to these when having a more informal stroll without a particular destination, length of time to walk for and a route that you make up as you go along. This can be quite freeing, too, and take away from the more formal approach of walking back and forth in a line. It might also be quite exposing to do that in a public place inviting curious onlookers. For that reason, walking a loop might be easier. See if you can find whatever is most comfortable for you.

The exercise I outline below can also be integrated with the other meditation exercises I have described in the book. Feel free to be creative in adapting these other techniques to this different posture. There's no reason why you can't focus on your breath or practice a body scanning technique while walking rather than the walking itself being the object of the meditation. It might be a bit more difficult to focus, but at the same time, if sitting is particularly uncomfortable for you, walking can enable you to meditate in a more effective way.

Pick a meditation path that is about 10 metres in length and has a marker at the beginning and end, such as a tree, fence or pile of leaves. Choose an area which doesn't have too much noise, where no one will cross over your path and there won't be too many people milling about. Pick a length of time for your timer which you think is attainable and where you won't be time checking to see how much time is left. Some people prefer to walk bare feet so they can feel the sensations of the ground easier, and this makes the situation more unique than a usual walk. Stand at the beginning of the path with your hands behind your back or in your pockets with feet about shoulder width apart. As you stand still, take a moment to ground yourself. Do this literally by feeling the connection between your feet and the earth beneath you. Become aware of your body and the breath that flows in and out, anchoring you to the present moment. If outside, feel any air movement on your face or body and notice any sounds that might be close or far away. Consciously put aside any thoughts about worries you might have or things you might wish to do. Make the intention to try to keep your focus for the full length of the path and take three sighs.

Begin to walk slowly and deliberately with your eyes looking a few paces ahead. Make sure you don't walk so slowly that you are wobbly and it feels very contrived. Equally, if you walk too quickly then it will be hard to remain focussed. Find a midpoint that suits you. Pay close attention to each step as your feet make contact with the ground. Feel the sensations of walking – the movement of your foot as it plants itself on the ground heel to toe, the movement of the leg and the rest of your body as it is propelled forward and how the weight shifts from one foot to the other. Feel the gentle rhythm of your movements and how they tie in with your breath coming in and going out.

If your mind wanders, remember to gently bring it back to the sensations of your feet and if you need some more sensory input, the breath too. When you get to the other end of the path, slowly turn around, take a sigh and begin the same process again walking back to where you first started, again with the intention of reaching the end of the path and remaining focussed on your movements. Every time your mind wanders, see if you can notice it a bit earlier and gently bring your attention back to the sensations of your feet with the ground and the rhythmic movement of the entire body.

As you continue walking, you can engage your senses, opening up your awareness beyond the movement of the body as you walk and breathe. Notice the sights of the path in front of you – the colours, shapes and textures of the ground. Observe the play of light and shadows, the beauty of nature and the details often overlooked. Listen to the sounds that surround you – the rustling leaves, chirping birds and distant (or close) traffic. Feel the sensation of the air on your skin, the breeze across your face, or the warmth of the sun. As mentioned before, you can also bring your attention to your breath more closely or start one of the many meditation exercises which have been outlined in this book.

Progressive Muscle Relaxation

This practice can be a helpful precursor to the body scanning meditation in the chapter on *Body-Centred Psychotherapy* if it is too challenging to get in touch with the bodily sensations on such a fine scale. It can bring greater awareness of the body by an initial stimulation of a muscle by tensing it and then consequential relaxing. This allows for a direct experience of the movement and sensation of a specific part of the body. If you are aware of a particular part of your body which tends to hold tension, then learning what it might feel to relax after actively tensing it can be a first step towards releasing bodily tensions that unconsciously build up. Typically, tensions help in the jaw, neck and back, but equally can occur throughout the body. Many long-term physical issues, such as back pain, can be tracked back to a physical tension related to stress, the body holding the psychic tension leading to potentially poor posture.

Find a comfortable position, either sitting or lying down, and close your eyes if you feel comfortable doing so. This practice focusses solely on the tension and release of muscles at different parts of the body. I start from the toes and work up, but you can equally start from the head and work your way downwards. I mainly have suggested this way of starting to show the opposite of the body scanning method described earlier in the book. Either work your way through each bodily section one by one or try each section a few times to become familiar with that area of the body, especially if it's one which is particularly tense or devoid of apparent sensations when doing a body scan meditation.

Feet and toes – Take a deep breath in and tense the muscles in your feet and toes. Hold for a moment, feeling the tension building up. Notice the different sensations that arise and change in the toes and feet – may be throbbing, tightness, some discomfort or pain, heat and stretching on the skin's surface. Now, exhale and release all the tension, allowing your feet and toes to relax completely. If it's hard for them to relax, try moving them slightly again and relaxing them to feel that difference. Focus on the new sensations that arise between the stage of tension and relaxation and how they change throughout the relaxation phase. Perhaps there is an initial tingling that then dissipates followed by another buzzing sensation. Compare and contrast with the phase of tension before moving to the next part of the body

Lower legs – calves and shins – Inhale deeply through your nose and flex your feet towards your knees, tensing the muscles in your calves and shins. Hold for a moment, experiencing the sensations of the tension before exhaling through the nose, releasing all the tension and feeling the muscles in your lower legs relaxing.

Upper legs – thighs and knees – Take a deep breath in and tighten the muscles in your thighs feeling your knees lock. Hold for a moment, feeling the pressure in your upper legs and the weight of your legs being held. As you exhale, release the tension, allowing your thighs to soften and let go completely.

Buttocks – Inhale deeply and clench your buttocks tightly. Hold for a moment, then exhale, and release all the tension in this area, letting it melt away.

Abdomen – Take a deep breath in, tense the muscles in your abdomen, and hold for a moment. See if you can feel not just the muscles in your stomach, but also the sense of squeezing throughout your abdomen. Now, exhale and let go of all the tension, feeling your belly becoming soft and relaxed.

Shoulders and chest – Inhale deeply, filling your chest, lift your shoulders up towards your ears and tensing the muscles in this area. Notice your chest moving upwards and outwards as the volume of your upper body increases. Hold for a moment, then slowly exhale and release all the volume of air out from your body, feeling your chest and shoulders relaxing. If you are feeling particularly tense today then repeat this two more times really focussing in on the movement of air and your body with the different sensations that arise in your chest as you move between the phases of tension in the inhalation and relaxation as you breathe out.

Arms and hands – Inhale through the nose and make tight fists with your hands, tensing the muscles in your arms and hands. Hold for a moment, then exhale, and release all the tension, feeling your arms and hands becoming loose and at ease. Repeat this with just your hands, trying to slow down the process to feel the increase in pressure and tension through each finger and palm and then the change in sensations occurring again through each section of the different fingers.

Neck – Inhale deeply and gently tilt your head back, feeling a stretch in your neck. Hold for a moment, then exhale, and bring your head back to a neutral position, letting go of any tension in your neck. Again, matching your inhalation with the movement into tension, repeat this by tilting your chin towards your neck before relaxing to the neutral position and then again, on each side, bring your respective ear towards your shoulder.

Jaw – Breathe in deeply and clench your jaw tightly, feeling the effects on your teeth and up to your temples. Hold for a moment, then exhale, and release all the tension in your jaw, allowing it to hang loose.

Face – Inhale deeply and scrunch up your face, tensing the muscles in your facial area. Notice the pressure in your eyes, cheeks, lips and nose. Hold for a moment, then exhale, and release all the tension, feeling your facial muscles softening and any tingling or buzzing sensations. Notice how each different area feels either one by one or all at once.

Forehead – Inhale deeply and raise your eyebrows as high as you can, tensing the muscles in your forehead. Hold for a moment, then exhale, and release all the tension, allowing your forehead to be smooth and relaxed. Try again, but this time, form a frown on your forehead before relaxing.

Take a few moments to scan through your body and notice any areas that might still feel tense. If you find any lingering tension, take a deep breath, direct your attention to that area, and as you exhale, consciously release any remaining tension.

Now, focus on your whole body as a whole. Feel the sensation of relaxation spreading throughout your entire body. Enjoy this feeling of deep relaxation for a few moments allowing your breath to relax in whichever way feels most comfortable.

Breathing Throughout the Body

This is the meditation technique which I use most in my personal practice as I feel it combines a lot of the factors which other practices include separately. There is awareness of the whole body, a focus on the breath and its manipulation to develop awareness and tackle the different obstructions that might arise as well as a more active process occurring to keep the mind occupied. If I have enough time, I will finish with a period of just sitting, akin to the exercise suggested for the development of *without memory or desire and negative capability* in order to dwell in the mindset that I might have created. If I have less time, then it will be a matter of developing whatever calmness and awareness that I can. Sometimes, I will combine bodily awareness in the way described below with a sigh. I find it is a practice which is effective for me to calm the body and mind and allow for the emergence of a more objective and robust state of mind that can respond in a less reactive and more analytic way, which is more in touch with and aware of my own mind and body.

The concept that this practice is based on can seem a bit unusual and when I first read about and tried it, I found the idea to be counter to my understanding of physiology and anatomy and, therefore was turned off from taking it too seriously. I have written earlier in the book about the relationship between the breath, blood pressure, physical sensations in the body and emotional state. Therefore, I won't dwell too much here on these explanations. This meditation is often explained using ideas of bodily energies and while many might find that relatable, I will write more about bodily sensations and the experiences that I have felt. I would encourage you to put aside disagreements about mechanism and focus on experience. I have found that doing this can open up the possibility of using meditation in different ways, with this technique being a good example. Due to the combination of a breath and body meditation, it is helpful if you are already familiar with the *body scanning* meditation or at the least feel fairly able to focus attention on different parts of the body and what they feel like as with the *progressive muscle relaxation* technique.

Start by taking three sighs before allowing the breath to settle in whichever way is comfortable. Bring your attention towards the entirety of the respiratory system following all the sensations that are occurring on inhalation and exhalation. Continue with this for a few minutes, mindfully bringing your attention gently back to focus on the breath when it wanders off. Try to breathe in a way which allows the attention to focus as closely as possible and keeps the mind in a good balance between being attentive but not agitated, and calm but not drowsy. If you find yourself feeling drowsy try to breath more deeply and if agitated shallower. Alternatively, you can try to extend the out breath to bring about a calmer mindset or extend the in breath to try to stimulate more sympathetic nerve activity.

So far, so similar to the *establishing the frame* meditation. Now we will begin to focus on different parts of the body and at the same time use our perception of the breath to relax and calm down both how the body feels and consequentially our minds. Bring attention to the abdomen and try to breathe in a way which relaxes any tension that you might experience there, imagine your awareness of the breath filling the entirety of that part of the body. As you breath in and out, notice if you can detect any differences in what you might be feeling there. Try to reach a point where the breath and awareness of the body feels unobstructed, smooth and relaxed. We will then continue to bring our attention to different parts of the body and associate the breath with that location by bringing our attention to both the breath and that specific part of the body simultaneously. This will help to increase awareness, decrease tension, and bring a refreshed sense of awareness there.

As with the body scan, we will systematically survey all parts of the body from the abdomen up to the chest, to the throat and then the head. Imagine that as you breath in and out, the breath is relaxing the body. You might begin to feel a drawing in on your skin when inhaling and a sense of relaxation and ease on exhalation. Notice the pauses between breathes and the effect on the body. When focussing in on the face a slight smile can help to bring in some of this feeling of comfort and pleasure to the meditation.

Bring your attention to your neck and then feel the flow of this breath awareness from the back of the neck as it goes from your shoulders down your arms. It is often easiest to notice sensations in the hands and fingers. Try to breathe in a way that these sensations become more apparent and increase the amount of relaxation and ease in your arms and hands. It might be that you feel the lessening of tension as with a *progressive muscle relaxation*.

You might also feel some tingling or buzzing to different degrees, as with the *body scan* exercise.

Return your attention to your back and downwards through your spine to the base and across your whole back. If you hold tension in your neck or back, try to breathe in a way to relax that tightness. Maybe breathing deeper or shallower, perhaps more rough or smooth, slower or faster, play with the breath to find a way to breathe right now which increases awareness and a sense of ease filling the body. Shift awareness through the legs and into your feet and toes with arms and hands holding your attention with your breath consistent with the focus on the body.

Once you have surveyed the body a few times and it generally feels more relaxed find a spot that feels most comfortable. For me, it might be the hands, the top of the head or the middle of the chest close to my heart. Try to breathe in a way that maximises the relaxation, warmth, tingling or whatever other pleasant sensation that might be there. Try to expand that experience to encompass more and more of the body with that sense of comfort filling up the body throughout each in and out breath. Notice how it can change through each part of the breathing cycle. See how much of the body you can fill with this awareness as if you are breathing throughout the body. It might be possible to scan through the body in one way on the in-breath and another on the out-breath. Play with the breath and see if you can find a way where your awareness is expansive throughout the body with an associated sense of ease and comfort.

Continue in this way and try to alter the breath to tackle any challenges that might come up. The troubleshooting section will go into this in more detail, but continue to approach the meditation in the spirit of an explorer and scientist and you will be able to manage difficulties through discovery and experimentation.

Listening

In the following techniques, we will direct our attention to using the auditory sensory experience as the meditation object. Likewise, the *Looking* section will use the visual field. What can be special about these meditations is that they can reveal aspects of sight and hearing that you might not have noticed or thought of before. Therefore, they can give a fresh perspective on a sensory modality and, in this way, can provide a keen focus as meditation objects.

When thinking about this in terms of faculties developed to be used in the consultation room, these techniques help to increase a capacity to notice different things as they emerge, but also to be able to sit with an uncertainty about what that might be. We cannot be sure what sounds or sights might come up for us, and similarly, in a consultation room, maintaining a curiosity and openness to what might arise within the therapeutic relationship is crucial as well as being able to tolerate the inherent uncertainty therein.

We can divide listening into external and internal experiences. The practice is similar for both. For external listening, having established the meditation frame, turn your attention to listening and then open up your awareness to let in and observe any sounds that might be occurring either from the external world where you are or from your own body. This could be the sounds of the room you are in, such as a fridge, air conditioning unit or the creaking of the building's structure. Notice how the sounds all come and go, see if you can notice multiple sounds occurring concurrently and how they might be layered. If outside, the sounds of leaves moving in the wind, other people, birds chirping, cars, planes and other vehicles. There is even some evidence that the sounds of nature opposed to an urban environment seem to boost cognitive performance (Van Hedger et al., 2018). The more you focus, the more sounds seem to emerge. You can also bring in the sounds the body is making, which will generally incorporate breathing, digesting food and friction from the movement of the body against itself and clothing. Again, notice how they arise and fall, how they layer into each other and follow these sounds for the length of time of session.

There is another type of listening where attention can be turned inwards to a type of inner sound. This is known by the Sanskrit *nada yoga* from the Hindu tradition where nada, meaning sound, points towards this inner high-pitched ringing sound that seems to be apparent during times of external silence, and yoga means union or in this context, meditating as in union with nada. The traditional explanation is one of some kind of cosmic sound that it is possible to tune into. However, it could also be thought of as a low-level tinnitus related to the absence of an external vibration in the inner ear, or a sort of auditory hallucination due to the absence of stimulation occurring. Whatever it might be, by sitting in a silent environment and quietening down the mind, it can be possible to attune oneself into hearing the sound. Then, this can be used for the focus of attention, like with external sounds. The fact that it varies less than all the other sounds occurring makes it harder to stay focussed on, but because of it being a constant presence, this allows for a deeper more focussed and less open concentration to be developed whereby the whole breadth of your attention can be filled by the sound.

Looking

I have suggested so far that most of the meditations be done with eyes fully or partially closed. However, it is possible to use the visual field in meditation either by keeping the eyes open to look at something specific, looking at something before closing the eyes or seeing what emerges in the visual field with eyes firmly shut. The focus can also be on something static or dynamic. For a static view, often people will use a coloured disc put in front of the face to focus on with eyes open. A candle is also used to give a more dynamic focus, the flame is flickering with the light moving due to wax being depleted. The eyes can then be kept open or closed and then the visual imprint of the coloured disc or flame remains in the mind's eye, either changing or remaining there. Equally, the eyes can be closed from the beginning, and you can notice what might be occurring in the visual field with the eyes closed. You might be very surprised by actually how much is going on when noticing the visual field in each of these different ways.

Another meditation technique I especially like is what I call *focussed noticing*. I find it especially rewarding to observe things in the natural world, such as a leaf, tree or patch of grass. By keeping the visual field static in that particular place, what appears to be just a leaf initially slowly develops into something more and more detailed the longer it is observed. Each aspect of the leaf's structure becomes clearer and clearer the longer you can maintain a focus and it can be quite extraordinary to see just how much is filtered out by the mind. If looking at a patch of grass the detail is even more so – what appears to be at first glance something fairly mundane becomes a dynamic, detailed and beautiful view. The diversity in shape and colour slowly increases, movement in the plants, visits from animals and depth emerge into an experience that can transform how you view the world around. It brings to mind the initial verse from William Blake's poem *Auguries of Innocence*:

> *To see a World in a Grain of Sand*
> *And a Heaven in a Wild Flower*
> *Hold Infinity in the palm of your hand*
> *And Eternity in an hour*

Focussed noticing is a helpful companion to the meditation exercises in the *Existential Psychotherapy – Working Phenomenologically* chapter. If the reader wishes, they can extend the processes of phenomenological, eidetic and transcendental reductions to objects in nature's surroundings as described in more detail by van Deurzen (2011, pp. 41–42).

Maintaining Awareness in the Activities of Daily Life

Just as walking meditation takes the practice off the cushion and into a mobile process, this can also be extended into those activities of daily life where there isn't so much of a cognitive requirement to be thinking about something specific to the activity. I have already mentioned using walking meditation while walking from one place to another and this runs along a similar theme of taking time that might be occurring in a sort of grey area between other activities, but extending it to some of those activities. This helps to challenge a sort of everyday mindlessness whereby we can get on with tasks and lose all sense of awareness in a kind of mental fog, seemingly continuing on autopilot. By actively maintaining some awareness or alertness in day-to-day tasks, it brings more focus to these activities, can keep us in a flow state and can help to shift our perceptions of self and awareness away from the head to the body. This will generally help to bring a more integrated and balanced approach to not only everyday tasks but also those associated to work and in our case, clinical practice.

A general alertness can be brought and maintained through a number of different methods, but generally, the idea is to bring a focus to a part of the body either while simultaneously occupying yourself with the task or at periodic intervals. Due to my practice generally incorporating the breath and body awareness I find that using that same technique helps reinforce the meditation practice itself.

If using the breath, then this can be achieved either by consciously taking a deep breath or a sigh and feeling the breath in all parts of the body that you can bring your attention to – the movement of the muscles associated with respiration, the changes in the body on breathing in and out as well as those other sensations that we have explored in other meditation methods. Having taken a moment to establish your alertness in the breath and body, you can then continue with whatever activity you had been doing, then if notice the mind wander away, mindfully return to the task and take another deep, satisfying breath.

Depending on the task, and if you have taken time to become proficient in the body scan technique, instead of taking a deep breath, you can make a scan through the body, or even incorporate the breath as in the previous meditation exercise. The practice might further integrate those functions developed while meditating into life generally and there will be an increase in focus and an ability to relax into whatever task might be at hand.

Inside or Outside

Being inside, the kinds of external distractions are expected to be fewer, although this might not be so true depending on where you might be. As mentioned already, if you can tolerate them, earplugs can be a great way to manage a noisy environment. That said, there is plenty of evidence that just being in nature has huge benefits for mental health and well-being (White et al., 2019) as well as cognitive benefits (Schertz and Berman, 2019) with potential improvements in happiness, a sense of meaning and positive social interactions (Bratman et al., 2019). For this reason, I will always advise anyone who might be struggling with their mental well-being to spend time outside in a green or blue space. Even if you aren't struggling but might be living in an urban environment, which can be somewhat detached from surrounding flora and fauna, it can be a good way to decrease stress and feel more connected with your surroundings. Therefore, if you can maintain your focus on the task in hand, walking meditation outside, or for that matter sitting can bring in these other benefits on top of the meditation itself. Managing the probable bigger range of external distractions it can also be a good way to increase focus.

In the Consultation Room

I will now present some ideas of practices you can do in the consultation room be that before a session, while in a session with a client, in between clients and at the end of the working day. Meditation can help in the transitions between these moments. While it is possible to bring these techniques into your practice even when having practised meditation for a short amount of time, the benefits will be greatly amplified if the other meditation exercises in the book have been understood.

Before and in Between Sessions

Depending on the therapy model you follow and the meditation technique that you find helps to support and develop the specific mindset you wish to embody then it makes sense to practise that technique. That said, time may be an issue especially if you are expected to write up notes in the minimal time between clients. For that reason, see if you can find a couple of different techniques with different time lengths that might suit parts of the day. There should be, for example, time at the beginning of the day for you to be able to sit and meditate. If it's a hard sell, given the accumulation of administrative tasks from other days, then you could consider how meditating can bring more focus and a way to destress, which will engender more efficiency in your work. So, even putting five or ten minutes into a meditation now, then you'll get that time back in the long run. Sometimes, especially early on in a career, there can be higher levels of anxiety before seeing a client, especially if for the initial consultation or assessment. At these times, performing some sighs, box breathing or any technique that you find especially calming can be particularly supportive for you to be able to approach the upcoming session with a more balanced mindset.

With the Client

I will describe the various situations where I find it helpful to bring a meditation practice into the consultation room. Depending on how you work, one might speak more to you than another. Equally, another may seem unusual. They are by no means exhaustive, and ideas may emerge about other methods that might suit you better.

Sometimes, it can feel hard to get a handle on where a session is going, or the experience with a client might feel in a particularly heightened emotional state. For many reasons, it can be helpful to recentre yourself in your internal therapeutic setting in order to reestablish your mindset and not become swept away by the situation. In these circumstances, I will breathe in such a way, be a sigh, or even just a consciously taken deep breath to bring my awareness back to one that is more focussed and return it to something more stable. As the breath is always accessible and a change in breathing can be subtle to detect, it is very easy to do this without a client noticing. Therefore, when I say take a deep breath, generally, I mean in a slow and soft way, rather than one which becomes performative or noticeable. This breath can help to bring me back into my bodily experience and the present moment, getting back in touch with the therapeutic mindset. It is akin to the idea of simply *taking a deep breath*. However, with an established meditation practice associated with your therapeutic mindset, this deep breath is imbued with the various mental factors developed while in meditation, including focus, resilience, increased awareness and attunement.

You can extend this idea to one where you consciously take up a deep breath while simultaneously experiencing the sensations that are occurring through the body. By taking a deep breath in such a way not just to increase awareness but also to consciously relax the body and mind can be even more effective than the above process. This can be a more challenging technique and is more possible once having practiced the *breathing through the body* technique. Once you have become more familiar with the breath and how it can be used to modify the physical and emotional experience, it can be a powerful tool to modify and adjust, as well as increase awareness of the body and mind.

Therefore, you can use whichever technique might be most appropriate for your therapy modality and bring that into the room with a breath associated with that technique. For example, if working more with a sensitivity to the body, using a body sweep either in a specific area or throughout the body can help you to identify or manage somatic countertransference. If working with an unconditional positive regard (UPR) and you wish to reestablish that mindset during a session, you can take a deep breath and experience those bodily sensations which you associate with that mindset. Using this particular UPR-related technique can be especially useful when faced with a client who might be very distressed to the point at which they may not be able to speak. It can be a challenge for therapists to know not just what to *do*, but how to *be* when faced with someone who may be in significant pain but is not at the point where they can express themselves with words or respond to the words of the therapist. Practising the generation of UPR, the affect itself and being in touch with the corresponding somatic experience, it can be a powerful way to communicate and follow those six conditions which Rogers proposed as being so core to the ways a therapist works with clients.

Having found a meditation technique that is most helpful for you, it is very possible, with practice to draw on that and bring your attention and that particular mindset with you. This is where the importance of making a home in the breath that I first brought in at the beginning of the book comes in. If you have worked to create a sense of comfort in a particular part of the breath during in meditation, then when you need to draw on the ease that might be present there, you can shift your attention to this home and find a place that might offer some respite from whatever situation might be presenting itself in the consultation room.

Reflecting on a Session or Client

As psychotherapists, there are plenty of spaces to reflect on experiences with clients. Some of these are more formal, such as personal or peer supervision, where reflection is aided with verbatim, process notes or recorded sessions. Others can be less therapy-focused, such as within a multidisciplinary team meeting or a more informal conversation with a colleague. We can also bring a personal reflective space into meditation and have come across something similar in the *Mentalisation-Based Therapy* chapter. By quietening the mind and then introducing a memory about a client or session, there can be a reflective space created. This doesn't need to be towards a goal of, say, figuring out what happened for a client in a session, or thinking about what a better intervention might have been. By making the reflection without a specific aim and using a non-judgemental attitude, we can see what emerges into that space and then again reflect on that and see what else might emerge. It is a sort of free-associative reflection and one which can result in themes arising that can either be used with a client or brought to a supervision for further thought with others. It can be helpful after a challenging session or when things feel stuck. It is especially useful when supervision might not be at hand and it can feel that there is not much space for thinking because of the challenging material that might have emerged.

The practice is a simple one. After a session, soon after writing up a verbatim or process notes, before or after supervision, or at any time when you can easily recall a client or session select a period of time with a bell or alarm and begin by *establishing the meditation frame.* Then, in your mind's eye imagine that client or session and abide in the experience waiting to see what emerges, continue this process, using mindfulness to return to the meditation object of the session or client when it wanders, as you have become accustomed to. When thinking about the client, try to focus on their bodily presence in your mind, not just what they look like, but how it feels to be with them physically in the consultation room and the effect they might be having on you as their therapist. Try to imagine being physically in the room, with you sitting on one side, viewing them oppositely. Bring particular features into your mind that perhaps you are struggling with. This could be an aspect of the client or session that is puzzling you, or an experience in the session that was troubling or seemed significant. Once the time is up you can write down what might have emerged in the meditation space you had created in your mind. It can then be possible to further meditate on these reflections and repeat until you feel satisfied with the material that you have created. This can be an alternative to writing directly about a session and offer a range of fresh insights about a session and the unconscious flow that might have transpired.

This idea of internal space for reflection fits in well with the concept of the *internal supervisor* from Casement (1985), the development of which has been discussed with reference to *unfocused listening* in the chapter on *The Psychoanalytic Stance – External Listening*. Casement also brings in the concept of a *trial identification* as supportive of the development of the *internal supervisor*:

> … I (also) try to put myself into the patient's shoes in his or her relationship to me. I try to listen (as the patient might) to what it crosses my mind to say, silently trying out a possible comment or interpretation. This helps me to recognize when a patient could mishear what I wish to say, because of its ambiguity or due to an unfortunate choice of words. Or, I put myself into the patient's position and reflect upon my own last comment. Frequently this will alert me to the unintentional, and unconscious communications that a patient could read into what I have just said. Then, when I listen to the patient's subsequent response, it becomes

easier to see when this has been actually provoked by me by my timing or manner of interpreting. I first learned to monitor the therapeutic interaction in this way by trial-identifying with the patient when following the clinical presentations of people whom I supervised. With practice it becomes possible to use these two viewpoints simultaneously, the patient's and one's own, rather like following the different voices in polyphonic music. This capacity to be in two places at once-in the patient's shoes and in one's own simultaneously-can only be encompassed if therapists can develop a capacity to synthesize these apparently paradoxical ego states. It is here, I believe, that the processing function of the internal supervisor comes to the fore. It is more than self-analysis and it is more than self-supervision.

(Casement, 1985, pp. 34–35)

This provides another manner in which it might be possible to reflect on a session or client beyond the visualisation exercise already proposed. It is less focussed on all the different mentalising perspectives than the *Adapted Situation Solver* technique in the *Mentalisation-Based Therapy* chapter and has more to do with identification and developing empathy. This method can be used in order to develop a capacity to occupy two viewpoints at the same time, first after a session and then eventually during a session. The trial identification can come in through a visualisation meditation, which creates that space to play, be creative and avoid some of those prejudices and previous thinking that can restrict more fresh understanding. Picking up where, at the end of the reflective practice, the client is brought into the mind's eye, we can bring in the client's perspective by again imagining ourselves in the consultation room with the client. However, instead of having what was our own view, see if you can shift the perspective into as Casement puts it, *the client's shoes* so where they are seated looking at you the therapist. You can then introduce the particular situation of the last session, or something that was said by you or the client. Experiment with the situation and see what it might be like to identify with the client in this way. You can also see if you can take a third position in this imagined, recreated room as an internal supervisor observing the interactions between yourself as a therapist and yourself as a client, creating the intersubjective environment of a therapeutic interaction and a consequential supervisory experience. When emerging from this visualisation it can be helpful to remain in a gentler breath meditation after what can be an intense and immersive experience or just take a bit of time to adjust back to a more usual way of being. A period of reflection similar to the first meditation mentioned in this section can help to see what might have emerged and consolidate some of the resulting thoughts.

The End of the Day

Once you have finished seeing clients for the day, there will be a moment when you transition from being a psychotherapist and shift your internal setting to a different mode. People manage this transition in different ways, often there is a ritualisation of the end of the day be that consciously or just by nature of the activities that always occur. So, for example, saying goodbyes to colleagues and maybe talking informally about the day's work, changing the seating or lighting in the room, putting any equipment away or turning off electronics, changing clothes or putting on a coat depending on the weather before closing doors behind and leaving the consultation room and building. For many this process is sufficient, but the nature of this kind of work means that often the projections of clients, the bearing and witnessing of suffering and the emotional involvement can accumulate and leave a residue of the day in the mind.

The suggested meditation falls into two parts. After having established the meditation frame, there is a visualisation practice to imagine the days' clients leaving the consultation room and, therefore, letting go of that accumulated experience. This is followed by a releasing of the internal therapeutic setting and returning to a more everyday way of being. This is fulfilled by essentially occupying an open, non-judgemental, present-moment awareness and then allowing it to be filled by the matter of our everyday lives outside of the consultation room. This allows us to segue into that transition from therapist to whichever role you might take beyond that of a psychotherapist. Sometimes, it can be hard to let go of this therapist's identity. I often hear of therapists struggling say when dating or spending time with friends, because others will feel they are with someone whom they are comfortable relating with in a therapist-client dynamic. It can be helpful to have a specific technique or process like this to ensure you can be slightly different in a social situation than a professional, given how much as a therapist, unlike other jobs, there is a requirement to be a certain way. I am not advocating for some kind of strong split in personality between personal and professional time, but rather a way to move between these different aspects of life smoother.

First, start by allowing the mind to settle, using the breath to calm down the mind and body as in establishing the meditation frame exercise. Then, in your mind's eye, starting with the first client of the day, imagine the client arriving and then leaving the consultation room. The visualisation of them arriving can have them open the door, greet you and then take up their position in the room. Then, without going over the entire session, imagine them standing up and leaving the room before the door is closed behind them. After having visualised this first client, then imagine the next, until you reach the last client leaving the room.

Once this process has been completed, then allow your mind to rest in whichever way it may find itself. Let go of focussing on anything particular allowing for an open awareness with a non-judgemental discernment allowing anything to come into your mind. Take a few minutes to dwell on, however, it might be feeling at this current time even if that means the mind turns to other exterior thoughts or fantasies. The idea is to leave your mind and body as relaxed as possible, without agenda or judgement. If you find that your mind is still racing with the day's events and clients, then you can take a more active stance – taking some breaths to relax or focusing on a particularly calming part of the body.

If your body is feeling tense or uncomfortable, then see if practising some body scans can alleviate the tension. Sometimes, a body scan starting at the tip of the toes and going up through the body and out of the head can be effective. I find it helpful to visualise a ring passing up around the body squeezing the tensions as if drying a sponge until they concentrate at the top of the head and are released from the crown. I hold most of my physical tension in my head and neck so find it helpful to do it this way. I'm conscious that you might hold more tension else-where and that other practices, such as massage, will always end with the feet to leave people feeling grounded. Experiment and see what works best for you.

Tailor this meditation to bring about as much calm and your attention back to your body given the amount it has been focus-sing on others over the course of the day. Utilise what techniques might be most helpful for you. This meditation will allow for some delineation between your working day and whatever you might be doing afterwards.

Chapter Summary

♦ Aside from the specific meditation methods described to support the development of mindset associated with different therapy modalities, there are many other techniques that can be supportive for therapists

♦ By practising the different techniques presented, you can discover which ways of meditating might suit you most

♦ You can also start to integrate your practice before, during and after sessions with clients in order to further develop your clinical work

♦ From here, you can work on developing which ways of meditating might be most practical and applicable to your clinical practice.

References

Bratman, G.N., Anderson, C.B., Berman, M.G., Cochran, B., de Vries, S., Flanders, J., Folke, C., Frumkin, H., Gross, J.J., Hartig, T., Kahn, P.H., Kuo, M., Lawler, J.J., Levin, P.S., Lindahl, T., Meyer-Lindenberg, A., Mitchell, R., Ouyang, Z., Roe, J. and Scarlett, L. (2019). Nature and mental health: An ecosystem service perspective. *Science Advances*, 5(7), pp.1–14.

Casement, P. (1985). *On Learning from the Patient*. London: Tavistock/Routledge.

Schertz, K.E. and Berman, M.G. (2019). Understanding nature and its cognitive benefits. *Current Directions in Psychological Science*, 28(5), pp.496–502.

van Deurzen, E. (2011). *Everyday Mysteries: A Handbook of Existential Psychotherapy*, 2nd Edition. London; New York: Routledge.

Van Hedger, S.C., Nusbaum, H.C., Clohisy, L., Jaeggi, S.M., Buschkuehl, M. and Berman, M.G. (2018). Of cricket chirps and car horns: The effect of nature sounds on cognitive performance. *Psychonomic Bulletin & Review*, 26(2), pp.522–530.

White, M.P., Alcock, I., Grellier, J., Wheeler, B.W., Hartig, T., Warber, S.L., Bone, A., Depledge, M.H. and Fleming, L.E. (2019). Spending at least 120 minutes a week in nature is associated with good health and wellbeing. *Scientific Reports*, 9(1).

10 Troubleshooting

I have compiled this section using a range of strategies and techniques that I have either learned about on meditation retreats, from teachers, other meditation manuals and through self-discovery. While it is the last chapter of the book, it is one of the most important as many people who start to meditate will stop quite quickly when they come across initial obstacles. I have heard innumerable times *oh I can't meditate, I just find it impossible to stop my myself from thinking all the time* or something along those lines. When starting meditation, just noticing this for the first time – how out of our control the mind really is, can be an important revelation. This is not the time to stop! That said, experiencing the initial discomfort in the body and mind when sitting down for the first time, not immediately reaching for a distraction and changing a lifetime's habit can be incredibly challenging. As mentioned earlier in the book, not being able to overcome those very early difficulties as a child meant I delayed starting meditation by many years. The support of a good teacher or group of fellow meditators is an excellent support for the continuation of a practice.

I hope that some of the techniques in this chapter will serve to keep readers meditating for a bit longer than maybe they have tried before. I think it's also important to point out that by taking a slightly different attitude towards obstacles to practice, we can disarm them from an early stage and prevent ourselves from identifying too strongly with them. By viewing difficulties as opportunities to develop rather than simply obstructions that need to be lifted, we can approach practice in a creative way in contrast to fault finding. This also halts them at a stage

DOI: 10.4324/9781003382959-10

where something more practical can be done. Instead of finding ourselves thinking that we are like the aforementioned people who just think all the time and can't do anything about it, or couldn't possibly meditate as there's no time in the day. Not everything in the chapter might seem that relevant to you, and to an extent, it can be viewed as a reference to be returned to if certain obstacles arise and support might be needed to be creative with a specific challenge. The strategies described are mostly to be employed in the initial establishment of the meditation frame section, although they can all be relied upon at any stage.

Distractions – Desires, Aversions and Doubts

We can think about distractions as those thoughts and fantasies that emerge in the mind while meditating outside of the focus which we are aiming for with the meditation itself. Three of the main categories of distraction can be thought of as:

◆ Desires – Things we want to happen or have
◆ Aversions – things we do not want to happen or have
◆ Doubts about what we are doing in the first place.

It is unlikely when starting to meditate that no thoughts or fantasies arise. In fact, in some of the meditation exercises in the book, these might be the desired outcome. But broadly speaking often when sitting down to meditate, distractions can be running riot and it is necessary to have some strategies to counter them.

The themes of desires and aversions generally fall into four main categories:

◆ Gaining or losing
◆ Pleasure or pain
◆ Praise or blame
◆ Fame or insignificance.

Mere awareness and noticing which of these categories may preoccupy us most can take some of the power of them away as they can then be analysed rather than feeling immersed in them. Some of the work might also be done in personal therapy. In relation to meditation, the point here is not to judge which might be good or bad, or be working in a therapeutic way, but rather to have some strategies to counter the distractions when they arise. In any case, these themes clearly have various biological and social aetiologies and purposes.

We have touched on how different ways of breathing can affect the physiology and consequentially affect in terms of calm and anxiety. However, if we look at meditation more broadly regarding the physical sensations that might be occurring, it can be noticed that not only are there pleasurable sensations, but also more relaxing and enjoyable experiences that arise and can be maintained through meditation. These ideas are explored more in the *body scan* and *breathing throughout the body* meditations. By enhancing these more pleasurable and enjoyable aspects of meditation, it can run counter to those thoughts and fantasies about desires or aversions. There is less space in the mind for these thoughts and fantasies if the meditation itself satisfies the parts of the mind that are looking outside for gratification and makes the practice itself a more attractive prospect. So how are these more pleasurable aspects increased?

As described in some of the meditation methods, there may be areas in the body where a more pleasurable experience can arise, often in the face, hands and chest. Physically, this can express itself as a tingling or buzzing sensation. In terms of affect, there may also be an accompanying experience of joy, happiness or even sometimes elation. Some people even find that their mind's eye becomes more radiant and the field of vision, with eyes closed, can become brighter. By focussing on these experiences and trying to find a way to breathe which increases them, it offers an alternative for the mind's focus away from the distracting thoughts and fantasies. With a continuous and regular meditation practice, it becomes more possible through training our mindfulness to get a habit of returning to these experiences, directing alertness to remain and notice them more clearly and being driven by our ardency to take up and increase them, but at the same time realise that dropping the thinking and daydreaming is actually beneficial. Part of returning to these experiences and focussing on them in a particular location when focussing on the breath helps to build up this concept of having a *home in the breath*, a place which can be relied upon to be a source of comfort at times when things might feel more unstable. Some meditation traditions teach to avoid focussing on and putting effort into increasing the pleasurable aspects of meditation as it may become the sole focus of the practice. I think this danger is fairly minimal as long as you use this part of the practice wisely as a means to manage difficulties that arise, establish and maintain more enthusiasm for the practice and keep in mind what outcome in terms of concentration and discernment you are looking to develop.

Therefore, we can breathe in a specific way, concentrate on a particular sensation in the body or affect, and focus our attention to build up these more enjoyable physical and emotional experiences. I generally find that a focus on wherever some of these more pleasurable sensations occur can help to stabilise the experience, combined with an effort to increase the physical area that it might have experienced in. Of course, this is not the ultimate aim of the meditation, rather, that is dealt with in the meditation exercises described, however, it forms a powerful technique to manage distracting thoughts that can overrun the meditation experience itself. This shifting of attention away from the focus on our thoughts and in our head, as if that is the totality of experience as a person, and into the body throughout the physical boundaries and range of different experiences helps to decrease the sense of being overwhelmed and ruled by this sometimes constant stream of distracting thoughts.

When it comes to the third category of distraction, doubt, it is the fruits of the meditation itself which eventually decrease it. Of course, this might seem like a bit of a circular argument, but it is part of the *come and see* attitude that forms meditation. You can read about all the benefits, positive effects, potential harms and any number of unusual and potentially outlandish claims. However, without practising it yourself and hopefully realising some of these effects in a practical and personal way, then the interest will always remain an intellectual curiosity. Likewise, the doubts about meditation, especially as it is an unusual activity that is often outside of the everyday things that people do, can often persist. Fortunately, you can notice many effects that can dispel some of the doubts early on. The moment you engage your breath in a different way and notice a relaxing of the body or mind, or even just see how the mind can often be out of our control and seemingly think of its own volition. These are early insights that perhaps can decrease those doubts about doing what might sometimes seem to be literally nothing. You might have also noted that I haven't put much of a time scale on developing a practice or being able to take up the meditation exercises described in the book. This is because everyone will be coming to these practices from a different place, and therefore, it's impossible to say how long it might take to be able to stay focussed on the breath for a few minutes or to develop a mean-ingful and fruitful practice.

Doubt can also come creeping in when comparing with others and having an expectation of where you might feel you should be. Therefore, stick with your own programme using the tips below to maintain a regular practice and this too will take away some of those doubts that can occur from expectations and comparisons. I will often joke to people on returning from a medi-tation retreat when asked what it was like that *I just sat around doing nothing all day*. At first glance, meditation might appear to be perhaps a pointless or mindless endeavour. However, those same people soon realise that when slowing down and removing those distractions with which we often fill our lives, while it might be more challenging, it can be a potentially satisfying use of time. Meditation is a curious idea in this way, but an idea and practice that has benefitted me and consequentially those around me immeasurably. By persisting and sticking with a practice, the doubts come and then go. A capacity for mindfulness, alertness and ardency borne from a regular and sustained practice will inevitably result in benefits. If not, then you will have just been sitting around doing nothing anyway, so you couldn't have come to too much harm!

Agitation and Lethargy

Agitation is the experience of being uncomfortable due to too much stimulation, resulting in anxiety that can be experienced often in the body as a physical pressure to move coupled with a sort of physical irritation, but also in the mind with a quick flitting between thoughts with a background anxious affect. Lethargy is a tiredness which again can be experienced in the body or mind but is not necessarily have to do with low levels of sleep, a postprandial lull or as a result of high amounts of physical or mental exertion. Like agitation, these can be driven by emotional experiences too. When occurring in meditation, if you stop meditating suddenly, things feel better, then it would seem that there's an association between agitation or lethargy and meditation. When put in a situation that is outside the usual habitual nature of the mind and it is restricted from its usual short-term satisfaction of sensory stimulation, there may be a reaction in this particular way.

When faced with agitation – try to focus on the drawbacks of being in that state of mind, notice how anger, envy and low mood can often run alongside it. Try to use the breath to relax by finding a way to breathe which lifts the pressure built up and brings more of a sense of calm. If it becomes too challenging, then you can also change the type of meditation and the focus, perhaps shifting to one of the more body-based meditation might help.

Lethargy can result in long periods of mindlessness. As with agitation, try changing the way you breathe, perhaps more heavily and shorter breaths. Extending the in-breath can be stimulatory by engaging the sympathetic nervous system more than the parasympathetic system. Partially opening your eyes and counting the breaths up to five before going back to one both give the mind more stimulation. You can also change your environment. Having a stretch, a glass of water or trying some brief exercise will help to refresh the mind and body. It can be helpful to meditate elsewhere or even changing posture to standing or sitting in a different way. I find that for me, walking meditation can provide the best response to lethargy.

Mindlessness

Mindlessness, the absence of the faculty of mindfulness can be perceived as a pleasant fug and potentially mistaken for concentration as very few thoughts or fantasies might be present. However, there is no alertness there and you won't feel refreshed when emerging from a meditation filled with mindlessness. It will be more of an experience of being unsure of what happened while sitting. Suddenly the bell will ring, and you will wonder where the time went. The key is to maintain alertness. Try to breathe in a heavier way to give the mind something to engage with. While it might sacrifice a level of calmness it will keep the mind from slipping into this lost state. Alternatively, walking meditation will help by making the practice more dynamic or one of the more active meditation practices such as body scanning. In some Zen Buddhist traditions, a meditator can put their hand up when sitting in a group and feeling lethargic. This request is then greeted with the slap of a piece of wood to shock the body into alertness. In some traditions, this isn't optional and if someone is observed as slipping in their posture, they might feel the slap of the wood to address this. You can initiate a more gentle version of this by adding periodic bells to a timer so that you can introduce a sort of external mindful reminder to return to your meditation object. This can work well if you find your mind is wandering a lot too. In Plum Village – a Buddhist community in France based on the teachings of Thich Nhat Hanh, a bell is rung periodically throughout the day for this purpose.

Pains

So much of our experience of the body is wrapped up in both the emotional state and attitudes at a given time. When asked to see post-operative patients in physical pain as a doctor, my initial approach was to make them comfortable in bed while taking some time to talk with them about how they were maybe making some connections between their worries and fears and their physical experience. Those who were more anxious inevitably experienced higher levels of pain and talking together, calming them down in the first instance, could often serve as an analgesic itself. A good clinician will first work towards explaining and calming a patient down before prescribing pain relief. Likewise, in meditation we can change perceptions and expectations of pains to alleviate their more uncomfortable aspects and also use them as a means to develop resilience and robustness. As a means not to identify too strongly with the physical discomforts that can occur in everyday life, from illness or as we will be thinking about here during meditation, I have found that calling them pains instead of pain to be helpful. The pain in the left leg can quickly become the pain in *my* leg, before *my* leg pain and then *my* pain. At that stage, it is intrinsically linked with a self-identity that makes it harder to disentangle and reduce.

As already mentioned, difficulties that arise in meditation can be viewed more constructively as potential teachers and none more so than pains. The acute, immediate and uncomfortable experiences are hard to get away from and provoke a whole range of emotional responses. That said, there are various things we can do to think about them and, through direct experience, feel pains in different ways, which open up opportunities to learn and develop robustness, resilience, awareness and understanding of the mind-body phenomenon.

First, it is important to acknowledge that there are physical sources of pain from injury, illness, wear and tear, which may inevitably be aggravated if sitting in a posture that is uncomfortable. Therefore, it is important to find a posture that is perhaps the least uncomfortable. As explained earlier in the book, it is possible to be creative in posture and there should be no association between a meditator's flexibility and a fruitful practice. That said, I have found having a certain amount of flexibility to be helpful in reducing pains when meditating, so I encourage people who might want to meditate for longer periods of time to try some stretching to allow for sitting in more comfort. However, if pains are arising that resolve very quickly upon moving into another posture or don't occur when say, streaming your favourite TV series, then it would indicate that there is some kind of association between your mind, the meditation and the pains.

If it is still overwhelming every time you meditate, then change posture every few minutes to allow yourself to practise for a bit. If you can prolong that concentration without immediately reacting to the pains, then there are a few techniques you can employ to examine and change your relationship with them. Try progressing through these stages, each one may be more challenging than the previous one because of the time you might be bringing your awareness to the pains. However, by nature of the way you will be using your attention, you may find them changing in quality and severity.

- ◆ Without changing position and thereby losing the opportunity to work with the pains, bring your attention to the location of the pains and see if you can breathe in a way that might alter it. Try visualising your breath as moving in and out not just thought your chest but also that part of your body.
- ◆ See if there's any change in how it might be feeling during the in-breath or out-breath, if you breathe more deeply or shallowly, does it change if you breathe with a more smooth or rough breath, quicker or slower?
- ◆ Consider how you might be visualising the pains. If they seem solid, dense and impenetrable, then they can appear permanent and it's easy to build up a stronger identification with them. Start mapping out the boundaries and intensities within the area that is uncomfortable. Is the edge strongly defined? Where does it start and end? Is there an aspect that has a particular intensity? Therefore, is that less intense area relatively tolerable? If there is throbbing, then is there a respite at the lulls between the pulses?
- ◆ You might find that by mapping out the edges, it focusses in and, therefore, becomes smaller in area. Or at least the edges become more fuzzy. Likewise, if they don't seem constant, then the pains become less dense and so there are parts of the area and times within that area when the pain isn't present. The definition of the pains in space and time then shifts from constant and in a specific place to in flux and changing location.

◆ In the same way as you might have developed the capacity to spread more pleasant sensations from a focussed area, see if you can do the same to visualise bringing in some of these more comfortable feelings from wherever you might usually focus them. For example, if the pains are in your knees and you have a modicum of those comfortable sensations in your hands, see if you can breathe in a way that you feel a flow of those sensations into your spine and towards your knees.

◆ Try changing your attitude to the pains and see if that can make a difference

◆ Are you finding yourself feeling victimised by the pains that they are directed specifically at you?

  • Do you need to take these pains so personally or can thinking about them as sensations occurring help to distance yourself from them?

  • Are the pains directed at you or occurring in your body as you watch them?

  • Is it even possible to locate a position of experience?

  • Can you notice a quality of inconsistency in the pains, which reduces the sense of permanence?

These ways of using breath and self-inquiry can help reduce the effects of pain in general. There are also some techniques you can use if you are specifically experiencing headaches that are associated with your meditation, as is not uncommon and can cause particularly significant obstacles. Again, as with other pains, there are common causes of headaches – hydration, effects of sugar, caffeine and alcohol, high stress levels and medical issues like migraines. I would urge anyone who might be experiencing chronic headaches to have them investigated by a medical professional.

That said, if you are finding a particular association with meditation, it might be worth trying the following:

◆ Many people unknowingly move their eyes as they meditate, especially if they are practising a body scan meditation or one involving different parts of the body, as even with eyes closed, they are looking in the direction that they are placing their awareness. If you realise you are doing this, then periodically open your eyes slightly refocus them on a location a few metres in front of you before closing your eyes

◆ Notice the position of your neck and back as you sit. Try not only to avoid slouching but maintain a neutral neck position too. If you find that you are holding a lot of tension in your neck then first gently move it – neck towards chest and back, ears to shoulders on each side, then intentionally relax before closing your eyes. Additionally try to focus on the area as you breath in a way that feels relaxing for you. It might be helpful to practise the *progressive muscle relaxation* exercise too either specifically in the neck and back, or throughout the body if you find you are holding a significant amount of tension

◆ Using the same technique explained in the *body scanning* meditation exercise, perform a sweeping of your attention from the base of your spine up through the base of your neck and then vertically up through the whole head and visualising the attention and sensations going out from the crown upwards. Start again from the base of the spine and sweep upwards again. Experiment with this type of scan and see if there's a way to change this perception of the headache through a flowing scan of the spine, neck and head

◆ Try taking some deep sighs over the course of a few minutes or practise box breathing. Both these breathing exercises quickly and significantly bring about a sense of relaxation and take the focus away from more immediate discomfort such as headaches.

Maintaining a Practice

This can be a real challenge to do over a long period of time and my practice definitely comes and goes when I think about the long-term pattern. I would definitely encourage frequency over a longer time spent meditating on fewer occasions. Some people find a data-driven approach to be supportive and there are a number of apps which will work as both timer and diary, offering you a way to track the amount and frequency you are practising. They also can give a connection with other meditators from around the world who might be using the app at the same time, which offers good motivation. I am often turned off from using these due to the gamification that these apps use, such as notifications or in app rewards to motivate. However, I'm conscious that many people enjoy this and you can also turn these functions off.

It is fantastic motivation if you can find a group to practise with on a regular basis. This gives encouragement from other's experience including being able to lean on others' advice and support. There is also something special about sharing a physical space with others while all engaged in the same activity. This is especially true with meditation and having a group of people sit in (relative) silence, which I find to be rewarding and profound. Many groups might have specific religious affiliations, but there are plenty of secular mindfulness groups online and in-person. One of my hopes from writing this book is that a community of psychotherapists with an interest in a regular meditation practice will emerge and groups practising together will develop from the concepts put forward.

While an app can offer a means to track practice, you can also write a physical or digital diary. This can be quantitative, but also a qualitative journal which offers up a record of experiences as you progress in a practice. Not only can it show progression, but also give motivation as, hopefully, it will contain some of the obstacles overcome and times that a technique has been truly developed and established. You can also list targets that you would like to reach and then when you might have achieved those. Try to set realistic aims or ones without time limit that you will eventually reach.

Writing a journal can also be a chance to reflect and connect the *on the cushion* practice with things you might notice occurring clinically. Perhaps there is an increase in capacity to tolerate a particular client's presentation, or ability to reflect in a session in real-time instead of waiting until after, or a greater capability to embody the given mindset of a particular therapy modality. Whatever it might be, by connecting the meditation with the clinical situation there is a recognition of one to enhance the other. Using the questions at the end of each meditation exercise in this book that are suggested when reviewing a meditation session can also serve as a jumping-off point for a written reflection in a journal.

I have often found when finishing reading a particular book on meditation, I am filled with extra zeal and energy, which can be a great thing. That said, when this dissipates, there might be a lull in practice. It is therefore important to recognise that developing a meditation practice is a long-term project and while there can be ups and downs in frequency, things can be boring or you might find some backsliding occurring, there are various other things you can do to maintain motivation. Even if there feels like there is no time in a given day to put aside for meditation, I still count focussed attention on the body or breath when walking down a corridor, practising box breathing for a few minutes or trying a body scan just before going to sleep as maintaining practice. Even though perhaps not lasting a long time, keeping up activities like this upholds a relationship with a meditation practice.

If you have a specific spiritual belief system or religious practice which you observe, then there are obvious connections between the meditation methods in this book as well as the reflective practices or prayers that you might already do. Therefore, try to make connections between these beliefs and the meditation methods that you might connect with your psychotherapy practice. By having some kind of integration here with your wider life and belief system it will serve you well to maintain a meditation practice as well as reinforce your faith.

By meditating more, you will hopefully find that you become better at maintaining concentration, becoming less distracted and generally being calmer and kinder. In this way, using some time every day to meditate will make you use your other time more efficiently and effectively. Those around you will also thank you, albeit most likely indirectly, for having made these changes in your life. If you are a psychotherapist, then you will know from your own therapy that you will never receive a certificate from your therapist that you can display showing a successful course as a patient in psychotherapy. In the same way, the fruits of your efforts in meditation are internal, yet also can be seen simply by the way you carry yourself and interact with others. In this way, the time taken to practice can be very well used.

Chapter Summary

◆ There are many challenges when embarking on and maintaining a meditation practice

◆ By employing a range of techniques, these issues can be grappled with through the meditation practices themselves

◆ It is important to experiment and explore what works best for you as an individual, as the process of reducing these difficulties can enhance practice itself

◆ Working with obstacles and managing these issues can give a deep sense of accomplishment and inner calm.

Index

For Product Safety Concerns and Information please contact our EU
representative GPSR@taylorandfrancis.com
Taylor & Francis Verlag GmbH, Kaufingerstraße 24, 80331 München, Germany

www.ingramcontent.com/pod-product-compliance
Lightning Source LLC
Chambersburg PA
CBHW061247220326
41599CB00028B/5556